HEALTH AND EFFICIENCY
A Sociology of Health Economics

MALCOLM ASHMORE
MICHAEL MULKAY
TREVOR PINCH

Open University Press
Milton Keynes · Philadelphia

Open University Press
12 Cofferidge Close
Stony Stratford
Milton Keynes MK11 1BY

and
242 Cherry Street
Philadelphia, PA 19106, USA

First Published 1989

British Library Cataloguing in Publication Data

Ashmore, Malcolm
Health and efficiency : a sociology of
health economics.
1. Great Britain. Health services.
Economic aspects
I. Title II. Mulkay, Michael,
III. Pinch, T.J. (Trevor J) *1936–*
338.4'73621'0941

ISBN 0–335–09913–0
ISBN 0–335–09912–2 Pbk

Library of Congress Catalog Number Available

Typeset by Inforum Typesetting, Portsmouth
Printed in Great Britain by St Edmundsbury Press Limited,
Bury St Edmunds

The virtue assigned to the affairs of the world is a virtue with many bends, angles and elbows, so as to join and adapt itself to human weakness; mixed and artificial, not straight, clean, constant or purely innocent.

Montaigne

Be rational; agree with me.

Anon

Contents

List of figures and tables

List of abbreviations

AIP	Agreement in Principle (see Ch. 7)
AMP	Ashmore, Mulkay and Pinch (see Ch. 8)
BMA	British Medical Association (see Ch. 4)
CASPE	Clinical Accountability, Service Planning and Evaluation (see Ch. 6)
CAT	Clinically Accountable Team (see Ch. 6)
CHE	Centre for Health Economics (see Chs. 1, 3, 4 and Appendix)
DGH	District General Hospital (see Chs. 1, 3 and 7)
DHA	District Health Authority (see Chs. 1 and 7)
DHSS	Department of Health and Social Security (see Chs. 1, 3, 6 and 7)
DMT	District Management Team (see Chs. 1 and 6)
GP	General Practitioner (see Chs. 1 and 4)
HA	Health Authority (see Chs. 1 and 3)
HE	Health Economics (see Appendix)
HEART	Health Economists' Activities, Research and Teaching (see Ch. 1)
HESG	Health Economists' Study Group (see Chs. 1 and 6)
IHSM	Institute of Health Service Managers (see Ch. 4)
MD	Mooney and Drummond (see Chs. 2 and 8)
NHS	National Health Service (see Ch. 1)
PACT	Planning Agreement with Clinical Teams (see Ch. 6)
PAM	Pinch, Ashmore and Mulkay (see Ch. 8)
QALY	Quality Adjusted Life Year (see Chs. 4 and 5)
RAWP	Resource Allocation Working Party (see Chs. 3 and 4)
RCN	Royal College of Nursing (see Ch. 4)
RHA	Regional Health Authority (see Chs. 1 and 3)
YHEC	York Health Economics Consortium (see Appendix)

Acknowledgements

This book owes most to the community of British health economists, whose members have been unfailingly co-operative and helpful. In particular, we would like to thank Alan Maynard and everyone at the Centre for Health Economics, University of York; Martin Buxton and colleagues at the Health Economics Research Group, Brunel University; and Gavin Mooney and the members of the Health Economics Research Unit, University of Aberdeen. For expediting our entry into the community so promptly, we have to thank John Hutton, organizer of the Health Economists' Study Group and Keith Hartley, Director of the Institute for Research in the Social Sciences, University of York.

We wish to thank all our interviewees for being so generous with their time and their ideas: Ron Akehurst, Joy Ashby, Dr Ian Andrews, Gordon Best, Dr John Bingle, Stephen Birch, Chris Blades, Nick Bosanquet, Martin Buxton, Dr A.S. Campbell, John Cairns, Roy Carr-Hill, Ann Coulson, John Cullis, Tony Culyer, Cam Donaldson, Peter Draper, Mike Drummond, Paul Fenn, Brian Ferguson, Graham Foote, Karen Gerard, Christine Godfrey, Dr S. Goh, Alistair Gray, Claire Gudex, John Harris, John Henderson, Walter Holland, Delia Hudson, Jeremy Hurst, John Hutton, Bryan Jennett, Paul Kind, Julian LeGrand, Dr C.M.E. Lennox, Mr J.M. Lennox, Graham Loomes, Karin Lowson, Ann Ludbrook, Ian McAvinchey, Alistair McGuire, Klim McPherson, John Marsden, Alan Maynard, Caroline Miles, Gavin Mooney, Colin Morgan, Miranda Mugford, Bernie O'Brien, Linda Oldroyd, David Parkin, Jenny Roberts, Dr John Roberts, Alan Shiell, Chris Spoor, Patricia Stuart, Dr Jennifer Tarry, George Teeling-Smith, John Todd, Dr Jo Wallsworth-Bell, Peter West, Iden Wickings, Jayne Wilde, Dr David Wilkinson, Alan Williams, Brian Yule and two anonymous evaluators of clinical budgeting experiments (see Ch. 6).

For commenting on our work we want to thank, in particular, Tony

Culyer, Mike Drummond, Alan Maynard, Peter West, Iden Wickings and Alan Williams as well as David Edge, Jennifer Platt and several anonymous referees.

For their practical assistance with the research we want to thank the staff of the Department of Sociology and IRISS, University of York. For consummate secretarial help throughout the project we are greatly indebted to Vivienne Taylor and Computype. The layout of Chapter 4 was done by Ian Taylor and the photograph of the authors was taken by Colin Clark.

We thank the Economic and Social Research Council for funding the research (grant A33250004) under its 'Science Studies and Science Policy' initiative, Phase One.

We would like to acknowledge the following permissions to reproduce material: from Gwyn Bevan for his diagram 'The Management Structure of the NHS from 1982' (Bevan 1984: 199), which appears in a slightly adapted form as Figure 1.1; from the publishers of the *Health Service Journal* for the photograph of Alan Maynard (17/24 December 1987) which appears in Chapter 4; from the publishers of the *Northern Echo* for the photograph of Nick Bosanquet (15 May 1987) reproduced in Chapter 4; from the publishers of the *Times Higher Education Supplement* for the cartoon about the Centre for Health Economics (27 February 1987) used in Chapter 4; from the publishers of the *Yorkshire Evening Press* for the child's photograph (2 September 1986) in Chapter 4; and from the trustees of the Mansell collection and the publishers of the *Economist* for the drawing of Florence Nightingale, the 'early efficiency expert' (26 December 1987), which also appears in Chapter 4.

We acknowledge permission to include versions of previously published material: from Sage Publications for 'Colonizing the Mind: Dilemmas in the Application of Social Science', *Social Studies of Science* 17 (1987): 231–56 (in Ch. 2); and from BSA Publications for 'Measuring the Quality of Life: A Sociological Invention Concerning the Application of Economics to Health Care', *Sociology* 21 (1987): 541–64 (in Ch. 5), and for Prof. A. Williams's response 'Measuring Quality of Life: A Comment', *Sociology* 21 (1987): 565–6 (in Ch. 5).

1 Introduction

How far can the conclusions of academic social science be put to work in the world of practical affairs? What difficulties do social scientists experience when they try to use their theoretical knowledge to solve problems in the wider society? How do they attempt to overcome these difficulties and how successful are they? These are important questions for many social scientists today. We do not claim, in this book, to provide answers to them. Indeed, it may well be that these questions cannot be answered, in their present form, because they ignore the great variation from one area of social science to another, the wide range of problems to which social science may be applied and the diverse social contexts within which applied social science may have to operate. Nevertheless, in undertaking this study we have assumed that social scientists in general will be interested to learn about, and will be able to draw their own practical conclusions from, the aims, accomplishments and frustrations of a group of fellow analysts who have accepted the challenge of trying to employ their social science for the direct practical benefit of the members of society at large.

In the chapters that follow, we report on the activities of the intellectual community of health economists in present-day Britain. The members of this community have regularly claimed to be committed, not only to understanding and developing the economics of health care, but also to the practical task of improving the provision of health care services in their society; and, indeed, there seem to be good reasons for being confident that the science of economics can successfully be applied in this area of practical action. In the first place, economics appears to be the most intellectually advanced of the social sciences. For example, it has an extensive body of coherent theory, its analyses are often mathematical in form and it is the one social science discipline whose members are eligible for receipt of a Nobel Prize. In these respects, economics seems to resemble the physical and biological sciences. We might reasonably expect, therefore, that its theoretical formulations could be used, like those of the natural sciences, to produce concrete, practical benefits.

Second, the period in which British health economics came into being and grew rapidly in size, that is the 1970s and 1980s, coincided with a general increase in the use of trained economists in government.

> Beginning in the mid-1960s the number of professional economists within central government increased dramatically (from less than 25 in 1964 to more than 350 in 1975). By the end of the 1970s the economics profession had come to be represented in virtually all parts of Whitehall, and government economists were engaged in work ranging across all aspects of the discipline.
>
> (Colvin 1985: 2)

It seems that British health economists' practical endeavours have taken place in a relatively favourable context in the sense that the general relevance of economists' professional expertise to matters of social policy was becoming more widely accepted within government administration and in the sense that other economists were already involved in applying their knowledge to areas of practical activity. In other words, British health economists began their work in a setting where the practical usefulness of economics was beginning to be acknowledged and where economists were beginning to participate in the social networks concerned with the creation and implementation of public policy.

In addition, the focus upon health care appears to offer almost unrivalled opportunities for the exercise of economists' skills on a grand scale. Government expenditure on health in Britain is very considerable. In 1985/6 the amount allocated to the provision of health care services by central government was £17,344 million. Throughout the 1970s and 1980s, as the cost of health care in Britain continued to rise, there was a growing concern on the part of government to reduce the rate of growth and to ensure that the resources devoted to health were used to maximum efficiency. Within the health care system, participants had increasingly to monitor their own economic performance, to cut costs, to rationalize services and to make difficult choices between alternative ways of spending the funds made available by central government. It was in this climate that the community of health economists came into being and began to contribute in various ways to the running of the health care system. Its members appeared to have a major opportunity to put their economic theories to work in the service of a crucially important social organization desperately in need of helpful economic guidance.

Despite the growing sophistication of economic theory, the increasing use of economics in government and the evident economic problems of the health care service, health economists have found it far from easy to achieve the kind of impact that they might reasonably have expected. We will explore why this has been so in later chapters. The point we wish to emphasize here is that few applied social scientists are likely to work in an environment as generally advantageous as that enjoyed by contemporary British health economists. While their achievements should, quite legitimately, encourage other applied social scientists, their disappointments and failures must stand as a warning to us all of the inherent difficulty of using academic social science as a basis for practical assistance to others.

The National Health Service and the economics community

This book is about the activities and experiences of British health economists. It deals with the system of health care in Britain only in so far as that system is experienced by, and depicted by, health economists. However, if the reader is to understand the problems of the health service identified by health economists, the solutions they propose and the difficulties they encounter, it is helpful to have a reasonably clear idea of the main features of the British system of health care.

Although some medical care in Britain is supplied by private insurance companies, the main system of health provision is controlled by the state and is known as the National Health Service (NHS). This nation-wide system of co-ordinated health care is financed mainly from general taxation and most of the services it provides are free at the point of delivery. Although the NHS is a nation-wide service, its organization is different for each country in the United Kingdom (England, Wales, Scotland and Northern Ireland). The formal structure of the NHS as it was organized in England in 1982 is represented in Figure 1.1, which is taken from a paper by the health economist Gwyn Bevan (1984).

Figure 1.1 is inevitably an oversimplification. Yet it succeeds in conveying an impression of the scale and complexity of the bureaucratic structure of the NHS in England. At the top of the hierarchy are the Secretary of State for Social Services and other ministers in the Department of Health and Social Security (DHSS). These officials are accountable to Parliament for the nation's health services. At the next level down are the fourteen Regional Health Authorities (RHAs), with responsibility for populations varying from 2 million to 6 million people. The RHAs are subdivided into 192 District Health Authorities (DHAs), with an average population of around 200,000 persons. Each District Health Authority is responsible for a District General Hospital (DGH)

Figure 1.1 The management structure of the NHS in England in 1982

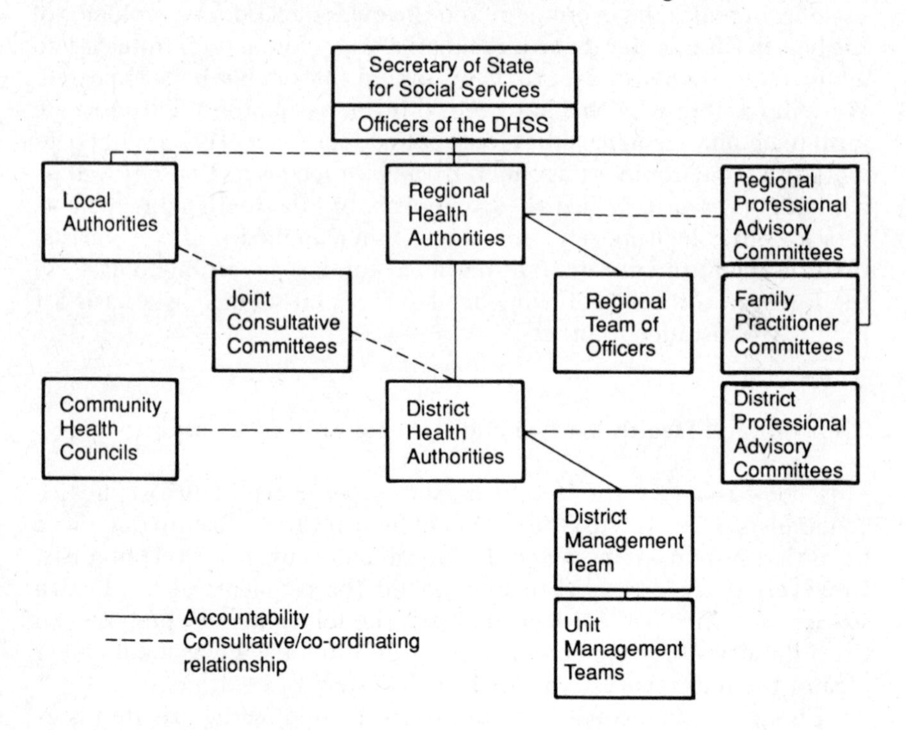

Source: Bevan 1984: 199

providing acute services, and also for services for the elderly, the mentally ill and the handicapped. In 1980 the number of staff directly employed by the NHS was approximately 790,000 (Bevan 1984). Family Practitioner Services have an administrative structure which is largely independent of the Health Authorities. Unlike hospital doctors, general practitioners (GPs, or doctors who provide a community-based service) are independent contractors not salaried employees of the NHS. In the early 1980s the number of GPs in Britain was approximately 31,000 (Dowson and Maynard 1985).

The NHS was established in 1948. The first major reform of the initial structure of the NHS occurred in 1974. Since then there has been continual concern over its cost, its efficiency and its management structure. A further reorganization occurred in 1982; and in 1984 the recommendations of the Griffiths Report (Roy Griffiths was on the board of directors of one of Britain's most successful supermarket chains) for wide-ranging changes in management, including the replacement of management teams with general managers, began to be implemented.

At the time of writing (1988), the NHS is once more said to be in a state of crisis, and radical solutions to its problems are being advanced which would involve dramatic changes in NHS funding and in the social relationships of health care in Britain (see Ch. 4 below).

The emergence and growth of the intellectual community of British health economists has been, at least partly, a response to the internal problems of the NHS. This is made clear in Colvin's (1985) study of the absorption of professional economists by British government:

> It is only in the last fifteen to twenty years that health care delivery has become a significant field of study for British economists. . . . During the 1960s in almost all industrialized countries health expenditure became the centre of a debate concerning the most appropriate ways to deliver health services. . . . The issue of costs facilitated the entry of economists into the health field in Britain and other countries. The profession argued that health expenditure could be more easily controlled if greater attention were given to efficiency in the delivery of health care. . . . Certain health economists found support for their work within universities and research institutes, others within government. Still others found sponsorship from private manufacturing groups with a stake in the health sector.
>
> (Colvin 1985: 145, 158)

The category 'health economist' does not have clear boundaries. It is evident that most people are *not* health economists, and it is equally certain that a few people most definitely *are* health economists, at least some of the time. But there is a disconcerting number of people who may, or may not, be regarded as health economists, depending on which set of plausible criteria one chooses to employ. We can be sure, however, that there was no *community* of health economists in Britain before 1970; even though there were undoubtedly several academic economists at that time who were professionally interested in health. Since that date an organized community has come into existence. Its presence is revealed by the fact that certain academic economists and others are now in regular informal contact about matters which they describe as 'health economics'; by the fact that specialized textbooks have been written and university courses established both for economics students and for people employed in the NHS; by the fact that research centres concerned exclusively with health economics, and funded by agencies such as the DHSS and the Regional Health Authorities, have been created at three British universities; and by the fact that the members of the community have set up the Health Economists' Study Group (HESG), which arranges regular conferences and which circulates an annual listing of 'health economists' activities, research and teaching'

(HEART). The 1987 edition has 111 British entries (Yule 1987). Of these, seventy-five were located in universities or other institutions of higher education and thirty-six within the health care system. These figures give a very rough idea of the present size and distribution of the community of health economists in Britain. They also reveal the dramatic difference in scale between the NHS and the community of economists devoted to its reform, and perhaps even to its transformation. However, this massive imbalance in size does not, by itself, mean that the economists' efforts are doomed to failure. For far-reaching changes in social practice have been set in motion in the past by even smaller groups of technical experts (Latour 1983).

The study and its method

In this sociological study of health economics and of health economists we have concentrated exclusively on Britain. Such an insular approach would be inappropriate for the study of most intellectual communities for such communities are normally international in their membership as well as in their analytical concerns. Indeed, this is true to some degree of health economics. Thus the HEART list of members in 1987 has fifty-six entries, about one-third of the total, from abroad. Furthermore, the theoretical literature upon which British health economists draw deals with economic processes of evaluation and choice that are thought to be cross-culturally valid. Nevertheless, despite these intellectual and social links with economists in other countries, the practical objectives of British health economists are intimately bound up with the distinctive problems of the British system of health care. As a field of *applied* social science, British health economics can reasonably be regarded as a distinct entity existing in symbiosis with the NHS. Because the aim of our study is to document what happens when a particular branch of social science is applied to a specific area of social life, it seemed advisable to concentrate solely, in this instance, on the British experience. Our general conclusions may, however, apply more widely.

We have used a variety of methods to build up our picture of health economics. Between 1985 and 1987 we completed sixty-five informal interviews with health economists, their academic critics and various health service personnel. These interviews were audio-recorded, transcribed in full and coded in detail. We also gathered various kinds of documentary material, such as research papers and books, technical reports, educational and public relations literature and newspaper cuttings. In addition, recordings were made of radio and television broadcasts featuring health economists, and of their public lectures and private seminars. All three authors attended conference sessions in which papers were presented and discussed by members of the Health Economists' Study Group. Several of these lectures, seminars and conference sessions were video-recorded. The authors also presented two of their own working papers to the HESG and recorded the presentations and the ensuing discussions. Finally, Malcolm Ashmore spent the first months of the study as an informal observer at the Centre for Health Economics at the University of York. It is clear from this account of the sources of data used in this study that we were greatly assisted by the friendly, albeit sometimes faintly puzzled, collaboration of our colleagues, the health economists at York. We must emphasize, however, that we interviewed, talked with, listened to and read the writings of health economists at all the major, and many of the minor, centres of health economics in Britain. (For further details of our interview sample and of our research materials in general, see the Appendix.)

One of our central aims in the following chapters has been to use these different kinds of data to show how the process of applying social science to the problems of the NHS is seen by health economists. We are aware, however, that our representation of this process can never be identical with that of health economists themselves; indeed, that health economists' own accounts vary in accordance with their differing positions within the realm of applied social science (Potter and Wetherell 1987). Furthermore, other kinds of social actors have become involved to varying degrees in the health economists' practical endeavours; for example, NHS and DHSS administrators, doctors, nurses, trades unionists, politicians and, in their roles as patients and as recipients of the mass media, ordinary citizens. Many of these actors see the practical application of economic theory from perspectives which differ considerably from those of health economists. Although we have not examined these other perspectives in great detail in this book, we have tried at various places to display the existence of alternative points of view by varying the textual form of our presentation. In so doing, our objective has been to communicate to the reader a sense of the interpretative multiplicity of the social world in which applied social science must operate and to convey that neither we, nor the health economists, can provide more than a partial account of the processes under study.

The threefold strategy

Health economists see themselves, we suggest, as the bearers of a unique expertise which derives from their familiarity with the principles of academic economic theory and which is, potentially, economically valuable. The mission of British health economists is to realize this economic value by using their expertise to improve the everyday performance of the NHS. In pursuit of this aim, health economists have developed three different, but complementary, approaches or strategies. The first of these we can call the educative strategy. When health economists adopt this strategy they attempt to change activities within the health care system by persuading practitioners of the benefits to be obtained by the use of techniques based on economic theory and by instructing them in the rudiments of the economists' way of thinking. This strategy does not require health economists to become directly involved in the operation of the health service, and may be limited to improving that service by helping practitioners to help themselves. However, it may also accompany or prepare the way for a more active engagement. The most obvious example of the educative strategy is the provision of courses in health economics for employees of the NHS. But the strategy can take other forms, one of which we examine in the next chapter.

The second strategy adopted by the health economists is that of direct intervention in the operation of the health care bureaucracy. This strategy can be undertaken either by seeking employment inside the system and by trying to influence specific decisions and general policy from within or by attempting to guide, advise upon and improve the processes of health care delivery from the outside, for example by undertaking consultancy work. Direct intervention is the health economists' major strategy. Their accounts of its effectiveness and of the overall level of success of their practical endeavours are presented and discussed in Chapter 3.

A third strategy which has become increasingly important in recent years is that of seeking to influence the activities of the NHS by engaging in public debate with other interested parties concerning the economics and administration of the health care system. The dynamics of this debate and the reception given to health economists' proposals in the public forum, particularly in the mass media, are the topics of Chapter 4.

Each of the next three chapters is devoted to a detailed investigation of a specific technique that is central to the health economists' programme of reform. The techniques which we have chosen to examine are measurements of the quality of life (Ch. 5), clinical budgeting systems (Ch. 6) and that form of cost–benefit analysis known as option appraisal (Ch. 7). In these chapters we pay particular attention to the ways in which health economists' technical procedures are designed to refashion the collective decision-making processes of the NHS in accordance with the economists' model of the rational, individual actor and to the ways in which these supposedly rational procedures are modified by, and absorbed into, what health economists regard as the irrational, socio-political processes of the health care service.

We conclude, in the final chapter, with a discussion of the lessons to be learnt from our study of health economics, with some general recommendations for the conduct of applied social science and with a considered appraisal of how far we ourselves as applied social scientists comply with our own practical proposals.

2 Colonizing the mind: dilemmas in the application of economics

If economists are to have any impact on the NHS, they must first persuade at least some health service practitioners that they are in need of help and that health economics may be relevant to their needs. Until practitioners have been convinced of the possible benefits of applying the principles of economics to their day-to-day affairs, they will not register for courses in economics, they will not employ economists in the health care service and they will not ask academic economists for assistance in solving their practical difficulties. In other words, the successful application of health economics depends on acceptance by, and support from, non-economists within the system of health care.

It is not surprising therefore that from the beginning, British health economists have devoted much effort to trying to convince practitioners of the usefulness of economics and of economists. However, it has proved to be unexpectedly difficult to achieve this initial objective. Health economists have been puzzled by the degree of resistance to their ideas within the health care system. The following quotation gives expression to this sense of puzzlement and to health economists' growing awareness that they must tread carefully if they are to succeed in breaching the defences of the alien culture of the NHS.

> Since economics has a real relevance to planning and can help planners with many of their problems, why is it that its potential contribution is not more widely recognised and taken advantage of by planners at all levels in the NHS? In short, what are the barriers? . . . There is . . . a danger that health economics principles are seen by officers and members to be too abstract and too remote from considerations of power politics and value conflicts.
>
> Furthermore, the culture of the health service may not make

> those within it totally sympathetic to the broad view taken by the economist.
>
> (Lee and Mills 1979: 172)

In this chapter we will examine in detail a public attempt by two leading health economists to overcome this resistance by medical practitioners to the economists' way of thinking. This examination will enable us to begin to appreciate some of the initial problems encountered by health economists as they seek to make their knowledge and their skills available to the NHS and to begin to understand how health economists portray their reformist programme in their dealings with practitioners.

Between October 1982 and January 1983, G.H. Mooney and M.F. Drummond (henceforth MD) published a series of twelve articles in six major parts in the weekly *British Medical Journal*. This is the most prestigious general-interest journal published in Britain for a medical readership. The series was entitled *The Essentials of Health Economics*. Gavin Mooney was the Director of the Health Economics Research Unit, University of Aberdeen, and Mike Drummond was a lecturer in economics in the Health Services Management Centre, University of Birmingham. The authors' objectives in writing these papers were summarized as follows on the first page:

> In this series of twelve articles we hope to provide doctors interested in health economics with an appreciation of some of the basic issues in meeting the objectives of health care within the resources available in the best way possible. It should also allow them to see in a fairly practical way what economics has already contributed and what economists and doctors together need to do to enhance that contribution in the future.
>
> (Mooney and Drummond 1982: 949)

Several pages later, MD provide an even more succinct formulation of their basic goal: 'Most importantly, we want to persuade doctors to be much more aware of economics than they have been in the past' (ibid.: 1025).

This attempt at persuasion creates a major interpretative dilemma to which MD have to attend throughout their text. In the first place, they have to convince practitioners that their present practice is in some way unsatisfactory. Yet they have to criticize participants without generating a degree of antagonism and opposition which would prevent them from getting the chance actually to put their knowledge to work in the practical realm. Second, MD have to show that health economists have command of a body of knowledge which is likely to be more effective, in certain important respects, than participants' own expertise. They have to demonstrate that health economics is more than a set of theoretical principles; that it is also a superior form of practical action. In short, MD's overall task is that of constructing a text in which health economists are depicted as the bearers of a specially valuable kind of practical knowledge which can be used to solve some of the major problems facing the health service – yet to convey this image without causing offence to medical practitioners. Let us see how MD cope with these difficulties.

What is economics?

MD choose to devote Part I (the first two articles) to answering the question: what is economics? In other words, they begin by defining economics. A considerable variation in the definition of economics is exhibited in health economics texts (Ashmore *et al.* 1988). In some circumstances, economics can be defined simply as 'the science of choice' (Culyer 1976: viii). In their first article, however, MD start with a rather different formulation, namely: 'Economics is about getting better value from the deployment of scarce resources' (Mooney and Drummond 1982: 949). Although these two definitions are somewhat different, they can be read nevertheless as closely related. For instance, the 'deployment of scarce resources' can be taken as implying the need for choice; indeed, MD later stress that 'choice [is] the central issue of economics' (ibid.: 1263). However, it is clear that MD themselves have exercised choice in furnishing their initial definition of economics and that their choice has significant consequences for how their argument is formulated. For whereas 'economics is the science of choice' seems to depict economics as a systematic area of study concerned with choices in general, 'getting better value from scarce resources' portrays economics as by its very nature actively involved in the specific evaluative activities of the everyday world. MD's preliminary definition, therefore, seems to be designed in a way that will appeal to practitioners in the health service and in other areas of practical action. An attempt is made at the outset to secure practitioners' interest by defining economics not as a discipline devoted to the abstract understanding of a particular aspect of the social world but as a practical activity concerned with helping people to do better than they are able to do without the assistance of economics.

Common misconceptions about economics

MD's brief definition quoted above is not, of course, sufficient to answer the question: what is economics? It has to be supplemented with further definitional work. One fairly obvious way of developing the initial definition would have been to proceed immediately to a specification of the ways in which economists could help doctors and other health practitioners to get better value from their resources. But MD do not proceed in this way. They choose instead to identify and correct a series of misconceptions about economics which, they maintain, are widespread. MD do not state explicitly that these misconceptions are common within the medical profession. However, this assumption seems to be implicit in their text; for there would be little point in devoting the major part of the first article to misconceptions which doctors did not endorse. Their procedure, therefore, is to furnish a more detailed account of economics by means of a critique of certain commonsense views about economics which are presumably shared by many doctors.

Thus MD quickly become involved in putting doctors right about economics. But they do this initially in an indirect manner, without openly accusing the medical experts they are addressing of economic error or incompetence. Medical practitioners, it is suggested, do have various false ideas about economics. But these ideas are not peculiarly theirs; they are, rather, characteristic of non-economists in general. Moreover, MD formulate their corrections in a way which shows laymen, including their audience of doctors, to have been at least partly right all along:

1. Money: 'Like so many misconceptions there is an element of truth that economics is about money. But economics could exist . . . without the use of money' (ibid.: 949).
2. Costs: 'That economics is essentially about costs is correct, but it is incomplete and subject to misunderstanding. Costs are important in economics but no more so than benefits' (ibid.: 950).
3. Cutting costs: 'That economics is about "cutting costs" is true, but it sells economics short. Economists are interested in cutting costs as a means to an end and not as an end in itself' (ibid.: 950).
4. Like accountancy: 'Both accountancy and economics deal with costs and both are concerned with issues relating to efficiency. Yet there are important differences' (ibid.: 950).

These 'yes, but' formulations allow MD to credit their non-economist readers with having seen part of the truth about economics and, therefore, as having some justification for their views; whilst at the same time enabling MD to suggest, gently but firmly, that these partial truths do a serious disservice to economics and to economists. In pursuing their definitional work in this manner, MD appear to be achieving two interpretative outcomes that are particularly suitable for this context. First, they are providing an alternative account of their discipline to that which may have been partly responsible for doctors' past resistance to economics. Second, by stressing the elements of truth contained in the common view of economics and by avoiding any open allegations about doctors' particular misconceptions, MD are rectifying these supposed misconceptions with a minimum of offence to their specific audience.

Avoiding confrontation

It is clear that MD are dealing skilfully with the problem of textual tactics that we identified above. Their text is based on the assumption that the NHS is subject to various economic ills and that doctors and others within the health service need economists' help if they are to learn how to deploy their resources in more cost-effective ways (ibid.: 949). At the same time, MD assume that participants' understanding of economics is incomplete and wrong in several important respects, and that these misunderstandings are bound up with participants' failure to respond enthusiastically to previous overtures from economists. In such circumstances a direct confrontation with medical practitioners is likely to be counter-productive. Any strong, unqualified critique of existing economic practices within the NHS is likely to meet with immediate rejection due to participants' presumed inability to appreciate the logic and advantages of economic analysis. Yet, somehow, the authors have to try to convince their audience, without engaging in outright condemnation, that the economic practices of the medical profession are less effective than those of economists.

In order to appreciate further how MD deal with this tactical problem, it is worth examining the paragraph in which the practices of economists and accountants are compared.

> Yet there are important differences [between economists and accountants]. For example, accountants will normally be concerned only with those costs which fall on the organisation for which they work, while economists take a much broader view of costs and incorporate in any analysis all the costs no matter on whom they fall – for example, the cost of home helps falling on local authorities. Thus, often accountants analyse costs only in terms of cash expenditure and not by the economic concept of opportunity cost [i.e. benefits forgone], which would include the time patients spend in attending for treatment. Accountants are

often concerned solely with costs whereas economists compare different patterns of use of resources with the various patterns of benefit arising.

(ibid.: 950)

This paragraph is by no means intransigent in tone. With the use of such words as 'normally' and 'often', MD avoid the extreme claim that economists' practices are *always* better than accountants'. Nevertheless, the paragraph does consist of a series of explicit and invidious comparisons between the two groups, in the course of which accountants are depicted as dealing *solely* with costs, which are conceived *only* in terms of cash expenditure and *only* within their own organizations. In contrast, economists are portrayed not only as employing a broader and presumably therefore more complete conception of cost, but also as being always concerned, unlike accountants, with the relation between costs and benefits. When comparing economists with accountants, who are not of course the main audience for this text, MD draw up a clear balance sheet which displays unequivocally why the economists' approach is to be preferred.

In contrast, MD's comments on the economic practices of medical practitioners are much less explicit. In the first place, there are very few straightforward comparisons between economists and doctors, and none at all in Part I. The main textual agent in Part I is not 'economists' but the discipline or body of impersonal knowledge referred to as 'economics'. For instance, we find that 'economics can contribute to the health service' and that 'economics is about opportunity cost and benefits' (ibid.: 949–50). Similarly, the defects of current economic practice within the NHS are described in impersonal terms and are never portrayed explicitly as being due to doctors' economic incompetence. For example:

There is an important difference between trying to economise and seeking out the most cost-effective policies to meet particular objectives.

(ibid.: 949)

Although greater awareness of costs can create a better climate for increasing efficiency, the question is unfortunately often posed without a real understanding either of the nature of the cost or of the problem.

(ibid.: 1024)

Often in health care questions are not of the type, Should we do this or not? but rather, Should we do more (or less) of this? Such marginal changes may result in very different costs (and benefits) from the average (an obvious point yet one frequently lost sight

> of). . . . Furthermore, the costs would have involved social intangible costs, which frequently might not be thought of as costs in the regular sense.
>
> (ibid.: 1024)

In these passages it is implied that in the NHS as in other areas of social life, people try merely to economize instead of devising cost-effective policies; they often fail to understand the real nature of costs; they frequently lose sight of obvious economic points, and they often fail to consider intangible costs. These failures, however, are not identified with particular practitioners or given a specific social location within the NHS. The formulations are designed in a way which encourages readers to accept that these errors occur regularly within the health service, without requiring readers to attribute them to any particular category of actors. Much the same points *could* have been made, rather more strongly, by means of direct comparisons between economists and medical practitioners. For the criticisms offered here are very similar to those levelled at accountants, where a more direct format was employed. In these three passages, however, and throughout the early parts of the text, such economic failures are not explicitly attributed to medical experts. The latter's economic shortcomings are identified only by implication. Indeed, MD's initial critique of economic practice in the NHS is not directed at the particular shortcomings of specific actors but at ordinary, commonsense economic thinking. MD's central message in Part I is that economic practice in the health service is inadequate because its members conceive of cost and of other economic phenomena in the everyday, 'regular sense'.

In this respect, their argument is quite general and could be applied, with minor modification, to almost any area of social life. It can be summarized as follows: ordinary actors operate with conceptions of costs, benefits, values, and so on, which actually prevent them from making the most effective and rational use of the available resources. Economics has revised and refined these conceptions, introducing new concepts such as 'opportunity cost' and 'marginal change'. These economic concepts, once they are properly understood, will enable practitioners, whether in the health service or elsewhere, significantly to increase the benefits obtained from the resources available (ibid.: 950). Thus economics is primarily a way of thinking about the world (ibid.: 1025). It is, fundamentally, a way of thinking which focuses on the opportunity costs and the benefits associated with changes at the margin. Economists can help participants to get the best value from their scarce resources by teaching them to think like economists and to base their economic choices on the principles of economics instead of on the tenets of commonsense reasoning. 'If the medical profession thinks of economics as something that only economists do, then economics cannot make any real contribution to health care planning and evaluation' (ibid.: 1025).

The ills of the NHS

After defining the discipline of economics in an appropriate manner and establishing the inadequacy of commonsense thinking about economic matters, MD devote the central sections of their text to explaining how health economics and/or health economists can contribute to the NHS (Parts II to V). Although the presentation of the case for health economics in these sections continually implies that existing practices are to some degree defective, MD attempt no systematic identification of these economic defects. A specific examination of the ills of the NHS and the economic failures of the medical profession is deferred until the end of the series of articles (Part VI).

When the economic problems of the NHS are touched upon in the central sections, MD stress that there is much room for improvement. Current practice, it is said,

> is bedevilled by the scarcity of resources, the difficulties in defining need, the problems of defining standards when little is known about effectiveness, the problems of meeting (and often only partially meeting) some needs as opposed to others in trying to ensure value for money in an opportunity cost context.
>
> In other words to ignore basic economic principles leads to inefficiency and inefficiency to less improvements in health than would otherwise be obtained. Improving economic efficiency can be a mechanism to promote less suffering and death. Most doctors agree with the objective but are less than wholehearted in embracing the mechanism.
>
> (ibid.: 1331)

Doctors are criticized openly at the end of this passage, which forms the conclusion to Part III, and their basic economic failure is made evident: it is their tendency to ignore the 'basic principles' of the discipline of economics. However, MD have already made quite clear on the previous page that doctors, at least in their role as clinicians, are not directly to blame for this failure or for the inefficiency which ensues:

> Too frequently in the NHS control over resource deployment is separated from accountability for efficient resource use. Clinicians are responsible for many resource allocation issues but they do not have budgets for which they have to account. . . . Clinicians do not deliberately go out of their way to be inefficient but incentive

> mechanisms and constraints are not there to channel them into more efficient behaviour.
>
> (ibid.: 1330)

The central problem, then, according to MD, does not lie with clinicians as such but with the organizational system within which they operate. Moreover, the defects of the present system are portrayed as having their origin in (ideologically based) decisions made in the relatively distant past:

> Until the mid-1970s much of what passed for planning in the NHS was little more than crudely based estimates of the need for physical facilities. . . . Perhaps the reasons for this are plain enough. A legacy existed from the early days of the NHS that, with a zero-priced system providing the best health care for all, the stock of ill health in the community would decline . . . and the proportion of the gross national product required for health care would diminish.
>
> (ibid.: 1263)

This idea that it is 'the historical development of the NHS which has encouraged a romantic' approach to economic realities is repeated later in MD's text (ibid.: 1727). Its effect is to displace the responsibility for economic inefficiency from the present into the past and to exonerate the present-day medical profession from blame. Thus, throughout the text, although doctors' economic inefficiency is often implied and occasionally mentioned openly, the responsibility for poor economic performance within the NHS is transferred away from the present-day medical profession onto the structure of the health system which they have inherited and onto what are essentially political decisions about that system made well in the past.

When MD finally mount their critique of current practices within the NHS, they maintain that medical practitioners have failed to 'face up to the tough choices' required of them at the national and at the local level; that they have failed to deal systematically with the allocation of scarce resources; that there is a noticeable absence of objective measurement of health output; and that the problems are 'compounded when some professionals retreat to the absolutism of medical ethics' (ibid.: 1728). Nevertheless, these charges are qualified and weakened in various ways. For instance, MD emphasize that 'there is much about the NHS that we (and most of our British health economist colleagues) admire. For example, we see no compelling economic reason to change the system of financing health care in the United Kingdom' (ibid.: 1727). They go on to acknowledge that there is 'much to be proud of in the NHS', and they cite a study which suggests that there may well be a general movement towards the kind of tax-financed, publicly directed system that exists in Britain (ibid.: 1727). Thus we are given the impression that, despite the inefficiencies noted by MD, the basic structure of the NHS and of the medical profession are satisfactory and not at issue.

In addition, in their critique MD profess to be presenting not an objective appraisal but only a personal view of the current state of affairs. Moreover, they accept 'that it is often easier to stand on the touchlines criticizing the players than to do better oneself' and they express the hope that they 'do not display the arrogance of which Engleman accuses economists, an arrogance which may be born partly of the frustration of having to watch the team's struggles from the side of the pitch' (ibid.: 1727; Engleman 1980). Finally, they combine their evaluation of the economic performance of the NHS with a somewhat critical appraisal of their own discipline and a recognition of the restricted scope of purely economic analysis:

> The aim of this series of articles was to introduce doctors to the essentials of health economics and to assess the contribution of economic analysis to solving health service problems. Nevertheless, the Health Service is neither totally 'economic' in its operation nor is economics as a discipline completely 'healthy' in its development. Both could show signs of improvement.
>
> (Mooney and Drummond 1982: 1727)

Placed in the concluding section alongside MD's critique of the NHS, the admission of the ill-health of economics serves to make that critique appear less pointedly critical and to redress any implicit arrogance by means of a humble admission by the critics of their own limitations. This enables MD to end on a note of co-operation and common endeavour, as both doctors and health economists are exhorted to work together to improve their present performance in pursuit of the same ultimate objective:

> In this article we set out a number of possibilities for change which represent joint challenges for the NHS and economists. . . . They are joint challenges in that not only do they require the NHS to counteract some of the sources of inefficiency already identified but also require health economists to enhance their own contribution . . . we see no conflict between economics and medicine. As health economists we try to understand the functioning of the NHS and see how economics can contribute to an equitable, efficient health service. We hope that doctors in their turn will see the value of trying to understand and apply the principles of economics in their pursuit of the same goal.
>
> (Mooney and Drummond 1983: 40–1)

Criticism without offence

We suggested in the introduction to this chapter that one major task for the authors of *The Essentials of Health Economics* was that of criticizing the medical profession and establishing the need for outside help without giving offence. We have seen that MD succeed in conveying, by open statement as well as by implication, that the economic performance of the NHS is defective. It is also clear that many features of the text do appear to operate to lessen the offensive impact of these criticisms and to reduce the likelihood that the audience's negative response to open criticism will lead them to reject the text out of hand before they have considered MD's positive claims on behalf of health economics. These 'defensive' textual features include the following: delaying explicit criticism until late in the text; linking criticism of the medical profession to self-criticism; treating explicit criticism as a personal and not a disciplinary matter; expressing pride in and approval of the NHS, both personally and on behalf of British health economists in general; adopting an apologetic tone as mere outsiders who are excused from the really difficult job of actually providing health care; avoiding mention of doctors as a specific group in the early parts of the text and avoiding directly invidious comparison between doctors and economists; using indirect, impersonal formulations when drawing attention to misconceptions of economics; focusing upon the economic inadequacy of commonsense thinking in general rather than doctors' specific inadequacy; excusing clinicians as such from blame for poor economic performance, on the grounds that the system fails to provide them with satisfactory economic incentives; and locating the ultimate responsibility for the economic romanticism of the NHS in various decisions made by the politicians of a bygone era.

We cannot, of course, know how these textual features affect individual doctors' readings of MD's series of articles. Nevertheless, we can reasonably suggest that MD have made every effort to prevent their audience from interpreting their text as a personal attack or as a rejection of the established, therapeutic ideals of the medical profession. Yet the aspects of MD's text on which we have concentrated so far are mainly negative and defensive. They convey to the reader that there is much wrong with the health service, despite the fact that nobody in particular is to blame. Much of the text, however, is devoted to formulating a positive case on behalf of health economics. We have already seen, for example, that health economics is depicted at the beginning as a practical activity designed to help other people to make better use of their resources. We have also seen that commonsense economic thinking is compared unfavourably with the refined and systematic principles of economic theory on which health economics is based. Let us now examine in more detail how health economics is presented to this audience and how the text works to convince its readers that health economists can provide something which is positively useful to medical practitioners in the health service.

Technical judgements and value judgements

MD's first step towards specifying the content of health economics is still rather defensive. For, at the end of Part I in which economics is 'defined', they raise what appears to be an objection to the very possibility of the enterprise of health economics. They ask: can economics be applied to humanitarian activities? (Mooney and Drummond 1982: 1025). A negative answer to this question would imply, of course, that the application of economics to health care was inconceivable, inappropriate or improper. We presume that MD address this question because it has been posed in the past by medical practitioners. Fortunately, they are able to furnish a strongly positive reply. It is obvious, they maintain, that economics *can* be applied in the evaluative realms of human conduct because 'it already is – albeit frequently subconsciously and in ignorance of some of the implications of doing so' (ibid.: 1025). This reply, brief as it is, contains the kernel of MD's portrayal of the positive contribution of health economics to the practice of health care. The essential contribution of health economics will be to make participants conscious of the economic choices that are implicit in their every professional action, to make explicit the underlying rationality of their actions and to provide techniques whereby such implicit choices can be explicated, systematically assessed and thus more rationally implemented.

MD recognize, indeed they stress, that the goals and choices of medical practitioners necessarily involve value judgements:

> In practice does not the Health Service, and in particular the medical profession, exercise considerable influence over the choices of resource allocation and hence of priorities? . . . Since decisions are presently being made on the allocation of resources, then at least implicitly values are being placed on the benefits of health care. Using the underlying concept of opportunity cost, we should only do those things where the benefits (advantages) outweigh the costs (disadvantages). Thus, if a decision is made to proceed with a particular policy at a cost of £x then implicitly the benefits are being valued at something in excess of £x. If the decision is against proceeding, the benefits are being valued at something less than £x.
>
> (ibid.: 1025)

Such decisions in relation to health care are unavoidably evaluative. They may involve, for example, value judgements about whether it is more important to provide better welfare services for elderly people than it is to improve diagnostic facilities for cervical cancer. But these decisions also contain significant non-evaluative, technical elements. Doctors, of course, have always emphasized the technical input of medical science. But MD argue that all medical decisions involve the use of economic resources for one purpose rather than another and thereby also involve, usually implicitly, assessments of the relative costs and benefits of alternative courses of medical action. The aim of health economics is to help doctors deal more effectively with these technical, economic dimensions of their professional lives.

In MD's text, medical judgements and value judgements about health care are portrayed as being primarily the responsibility of the medical profession. Health economists will, of course, have values of their own. But these should not be allowed to influence their policy recommendations (ibid.: 1405). When the health economist needs to know what the relevant medical and value judgements are, in order to give advice about alternative courses of action, he or she will necessarily turn to the medical profession. 'This implies again asking the right questions, and of the right people. Because of their influence over individual treatments and resource deployment, this includes asking individual members of the medical profession' (ibid.: 1486). The technical task of the health economist, or of any practitioner attempting to apply the principles of economics to health care, is to translate the various evaluations and judgements of appropriate others about various possible courses of action into a common framework for assessment and choice. Cost–benefit analysis and other similar techniques are used for this purpose (ibid.: 1562).

The input of health economics, then, is in principle technical rather than evaluative. Nevertheless, MD argue enthusiastically for the adoption of the methods of health economics because they will assist medical practitioners to attain *their* values more effectively.

> The logic of this simple approach of bringing together cost and output data to help assess priorities would seem difficult to deny, bearing in mind as always that costs here are forgone benefits. It is an explicit recognition of what most NHS personnel would accept implicitly – that an important goal of health care is to try to maximise the benefit from the limited resources available. Economists are thus not the desiccated calculating machines of Nye Bevan's portrayal. They are not attempting to remove the need for value judgements or even emotionalism in health care but are trying to provide a framework within which these can be articulated constructively.
>
> (ibid.: 1329)

According to MD's account, the existing system of health care is irrational, not in the sense that it involves judgements of value, but in the sense that pursuit of these values is undertaken in ignorance of, and without careful appraisal of, the full range of possible costs and benefits. Health economics is offered as a way of thinking and as a set of techniques which will raise the level of rationality:

> Economics can only be decision aiding and not decision making, since health care planning and policy making are inevitably subjective. Being aware of that and making the necessary trade-offs explicitly and hence more rationally is the function of economics.
> (ibid.: 1405)

Thus health economics, as presented in MD's text, avoids encroaching on the medical or evaluative responsibilities of the medical profession. It is, indeed, merely a way of enabling practitioners to do more successfully what they already (want to) do. MD make it clear that the methods of health economics are urgently needed in the NHS. Yet health economics appears to have no substantive implications for the organization of health care, beyond those contained in medical practitioners' own views and value judgements. Even the economists' central concepts and procedures are treated as already implicit in participants' choices. The basic logic of health economics 'is an explicit recognition of what most NHS personnel would accept implicitly' (ibid.: 1329).

MD appear, then, to be proposing a subordinate position for health economists owing to the purely technical character of their knowledge and their skills. Health economists are portrayed, in many parts of the text, as no more than modest technicians, who leave the important decisions to others and who merely assist others to make their choices more carefully. Health economics itself is no more than a set of 'decision-aiding' devices. Yet, in many other passages, MD appear to refuse to grant non-economists the right to think about their choices in any terms other than those of economics. The logic of health economists' analysis is said to be 'difficult to deny' (ibid.) and, even more strongly, 'undeniable' (ibid.: 1561). Whilst participants' actions are understood as entailing an underlying economic logic, participants' own attempts to explicate and implement this logic are regularly portrayed as poor and incomplete (ibid.: 950, 1329, 1727). The concept of 'opportunity cost' is depicted as 'inescapable' (ibid.: 1330) and is used time and again to reveal the 'inadequacy' of existing practice within the NHS (ibid.: 950, 1263). At no point is it allowed in MD's text that medical practitioners, or other non-economists, might not be governed by the constraints of opportunity cost as conceived by economists or that they might have a different but equally valid conception of economic rationality. To consider such possibilities would be to attempt to deny the undeniable; it would be to try to escape the inescapable.

In other words, MD's text continually asserts that economists' concepts alone properly capture the underlying economic realities of participants' social world. For MD, opportunity costs, assessments of cost–benefit ratios and marginal choices are constantly operative in the world of medical care, whether participants are aware of them or not. Furthermore, participants' choices are undoubtedly governed by the principles of rationality enunciated by economists, whether the former are aware of it or not. Unfortunately, from the economists' point of view, participants are not, on the whole, conscious of the economic processes which dominate so much of their lives. As a result, they regularly fail to implement the requirements of their own rationality. Out of ignorance, they fail to make the best use, in their own terms, of the available resources. It is here, as we have seen, that MD and their colleagues offer help. They cannot change the underlying economic reality of scarcity and opportunity cost; for this is unavoidable. Nor can they change the principle of rational choice; for this is universal. But they can help participants to become more aware of the parameters of choice identified by economic theory and how these parameters can be measured in particular instances. In this way, they can assist practitioners more fully to realize their own aims.

However, the paradox of this view of the relationship between economic theory and participants' action is that participants are deemed to be acting fully rationally, and are regarded as capable of achieving their *own* values most effectively, only in so far as they come to think and act like economists. Although MD tend to depict economists as technicians, their ultimate objective as *social* technicians is to transform participants, as far as possible, into economists. As MD emphasize throughout their text, they are trying to pass on to medical practitioners a logic, a doctrine, a way of thinking. As they state in their closing remarks:

> As economists our biggest challenge is in trying to gain wider acceptance by doctors and other NHS professionals of the ideas put forward in this series. . . . As health economists we try to understand the functioning of the NHS and see how economics can contribute to an equitable, efficient health service. We hope that doctors in their turn will see the value of trying to understand and apply the principles of economics in their pursuit of the same goal.
> (Mooney and Drummond 1983: 41)

MD do not propose, of course, that health practitioners should become indistinguishable from health economists or that they should abandon their medical expertise. They do insist, however, that practitioners should think and act like economists when they are dealing with the economic dimensions of their work. Moreover, given that economics is involved in *all* choices, and that economic procedures can be applied in principle to *all* costs and benefits, the need for a wide-ranging transformation of practitioners' thinking and conduct is clearly implied. Implicit, therefore, in economists' proposals is what we have called a 'colonization of the mind' (for a discussion of 'economic imperalism', see Culyer 1981). In recommending the widespread application of the principles of economics, economists claim to be offering practitioners the opportunity of realizing their own values more fully and effectively. In order to do this, however, practitioners will have to come to think and act like economists, whose view of the world they can no longer afford to reject as alien and as inimical to their personal and professional values.

The dual programme of health economics

In the earlier sections of this chapter we suggested that MD's critique of the medical profession was characterized by an interpretative duality. On the one hand, MD emphasized that the NHS was economically defective in various respects and that its performance could be improved significantly with the help of health economists. Yet, at the same time, they avoided blaming the medical profession in any direct manner, they expressed pride in the achievements of the NHS and they drew attention to their own limitations and to the necessity for active co-operation. We then examined MD's account of the nature of health economics and their proposals for using health economics to improve the British system of health care. We have found a similar interpretative duality here. In many parts of MD's text, health economics is depicted as no more than a technical aid that will help participants improve their economic performance without encroaching upon their medical or evaluative prerogatives. Yet, at the same time, MD continually assert the ability of health economists to identify the underlying economic realities of the health service, whatever practitioners' understanding of those realities may be; and they persistently propose that the health service will operate effectively only in so far as participants adopt the economists' way of thinking.

In the discussion so far we have distinguished, for purposes of presentation, between MD's appraisal of the medical profession and their account of health economics. But in MD's text these two themes continually intertwine, and the two dualities merge into a sustained interpretative movement between two versions of the relationship between economics and the system of health care. One version of this relationship, which we may call the 'weak programme' for health economics, maintains that the NHS has many problems, but that it also has many achievements (see Chubin and Restivo 1983). It is proposed that health economics can be of assistance to the medical profession. But it is stressed that 'the economists' approach represents just one way of looking at the world' (Mooney and Drummond 1983: 40). Within this version of health economics, the economist is essentially a technician, a skilled subordinate, a source of techniques that will help practitioners to attain their goals more effectively. There is no need for economists to attempt to influence or direct the health care system in any substantive way. For the principles of economics are already implicit in participants' own actions. The explicit adoption of these principles by practitioners will simply enable them to implement their own evaluative preferences, as far as this is realistically possible in an imperfect world.

In contrast, the 'strong programme' for health economics maintains that economic inefficiency pervades the NHS at all levels; partly owing to the nature of the system, but also as a result of practitioners' factual ignorance and, most important of all, their lack of familiarity with the principles of economics. According to this programme, health economists operating both inside and outside the system can help to improve things here and there. But wholesale improvement will be possible only by means of extensive training schemes. NHS managers, practising clinicians and medical students must all be trained thoroughly in economics (ibid.: 41). All practitioners within the health service must be taught to deal with economic issues as would economists themselves. This should be a major goal of the NHS, for only by moving towards realization of this goal can a truly rational system of health care be created. Health economists, as the most qualified experts in economic thought, would of course play the major role in guiding the NHS towards this state of rationality. It is the strong programme which implies the need for 'colonizing the mind' of existing practitioners.

These, then, are the two programmes for health economics available in MD's text. We do not mean to suggest, however, that they are separate components of that text. In *The Essentials of Health Economics*, both elements are inextricably linked. In this respect, it is no different from many other texts which depend upon, and generate much of their interpretative work through, the combination of contrasting elements (Atkinson 1984). Indeed, in the light of our reading of MD's text, we can ask what is being accomplished by the combined presentation of the strong and the weak programmes. As a first step in answering this question we suggest that the strong programme is essentially a restatement of the discourse of economic theory as it has developed within the community of economists, whilst the weak programme is addressed to, and designed for the requirements of, non-economists.

Theorists in economics strive, like those in other scientific disciplines, to identify among themselves the regularities which lie behind the diverse appearances of the everyday world. Like other social scientists, economic theorists look beyond the crude and ill-informed surmises of ordinary participants. But unlike most other social scientists, economists have been remarkably successful, in their own terms, in replacing such commonsense ideas with a set of elegant principles which have come to be treated by economists as the underlying reality. Health economics is often defined as the application of these principles to the field of health (Klarman 1965: 1). As one leading British health economist has written:

> Health economics as a discipline does not exist independently of economics as a discipline: there are few techniques of economic analysis that are not applicable to the topic of health; moreover, there are few theoretical ideas in health economics that are truly sui generis.
>
> (Culyer 1981: 4)

Such theoretical concepts as 'marginality' and 'opportunity cost', formulated by economists for economists with little reference to empirical observation, are none the less deemed to be universally applicable (Whitley 1986). They are used not only to describe and explain how participants do in fact behave economically but also, and perhaps more importantly, to furnish standards of rational conduct. It is assumed that *rational* actors *must* choose those courses of action which follow from the principles of economic theory – as long as they have full knowledge of the implications of their actions. It is of course accepted that, in practice, actors seldom have such knowledge. Thus economic theorists expect to find significant divergences between ideal and actual economic activity. It is recognized that 'economics' involves an abstraction from the more complex world of reality, where economic processes are seriously affected by other social and political factors. From the perspective of economic theory, however, these factors interfere with the requirements of economic rationality. Thus a major implication of economic theory, conceived in isolation from the diversity of actual economic practices, is that economic conduct in the real world can always be improved by drawing participants' attention to the principles of economics and by revealing to participants the economic 'realities' implicit in their acts of choice. There is, we suggest, an 'economic imperialism' built into the universalistic claims of economic theory and into its denial of the relevance of alternative economic rationalities. The strong programme in health economics follows directly from this form of theoretical discourse which is intellectually dominant within the community of economists (Colvin 1985; Whitley 1986). This programme is a direct reformulation of the literary practice of economic theory (see McCloskey, 1985).

When economists seek to enter the realm of practical action, however, as most health economists have done, this form of discourse will often be seen by recipients as threatening, as presumptuous and as intellectually arrogant. For it will seem to imply that outsiders are claiming to be able to understand more fully and to deal more effectively with the complexities of specific areas of practical action than those who have devoted their professional lives to those domains of social life. As MD comment, when the health economist visits the doctor s/he is likely to be asked 'with a wry grin', 'You're the health economist; which one [of two treatments] should I prescribe?' (Mooney and Drummond 1982: 1638). In such practical contexts the economist, if s/he is to get a hearing at all and is to elicit something other than a wry grin, will have to adapt to the values and to the organizational dominance of practitioners. S/he will have to emphasize that his or her economic structures should not be taken personally, that there is much to admire in existing practices and that, of course, health economists have much to learn before they can make a useful contribution. Thus, we suggest, the weak programme arises as a result of economists' entry into the practical context. It can be seen as a series of modifications, reservations and disclaimers designed to enable economists to circumvent the resistance created among practitioners in response to the challenging assertions of the strong programme. It is, however, this latter programme which provides the intellectual impetus behind health economics and which furnishes the theoretical basis for its practical recommendations. For it is the strong programme which stems most directly from the internal practices of the discipline of economics. Accordingly, although the weak programme is a necessary part of health economists' practical strategy in certain contexts, it is unlikely that the strong programme can ever be abandoned; hence the interpretative duality of *The Essentials of Health Economics*.

In this chapter we have observed the kind of textual manoeuvres that are likely to be employed when health economists directly approach the members of the powerful medical profession. We have seen that, in these circumstances, health economists tend to avoid open criticism of medical practitioners, to stress the convergence of interests between doctors and economists, and to present the economist's role as essentially that of helping doctors to achieve their own ends. In other situations, however, particularly where third parties are involved, health economists are often much less restrained in their enthusiastic advocacy of alternative economic policies and in their condemnation of doctors' economic incompetence. Indeed, certain leading health economists are said to specialize in what participants term 'doctor-bashing'. But this more vigorous expression of the health economists' strong programme is normally used to convince people who are not themselves doctors. We will see some doctor-bashing in Chapter 4, when we show how health economists have contributed to the public debate over health care. Before that, however, we will examine how economists have fared in their attempts to change the NHS by means of direct intervention.

3 Quick and dirty: the problems of intervention

Over the years, as we saw in Chapter 1, health economists have gained a footing within the British health care system and they now contribute regularly to its day-to-day operation. They do so either by entering the health service and trying to raise levels of economic rationality from the inside or by furnishing expert guidance from university departments of economics or from associated centres of health economics. In this chapter we will examine the accounts given in interviews by health economists and others of the major difficulties encountered by economists in their attempts to intervene directly in this area of practical action. We will also consider respondents' estimates of how far economists have succeeded in fostering greater rationality within the system of health care.

The interviews that we carried out with administrators, health care personnel and health economists contain far too much relevant material to be presented in full in this chapter (see the Appendix). We have been forced, therefore, to select just one or two exemplary quotations from the interview transcripts in order to illustrate and document each major point to be made in the following sections. The discussion focuses, however, on views that were expressed time and again during the interviews. We will keep our own commentary to a minimum in this chapter in order to allow the health economists, as far as possible, to tell of their difficulties, successes and failures in their own words.

When examining quotations from interviews, readers need to have some idea of who is speaking in each instance. It would, however, make our presentation cumbersome and distracting if we were to furnish detailed background information for every quoted passage. We have tried to solve this problem by dividing respondents into three broad categories. We have used the term 'practitioner' to refer to people who work within the system of health care but who have no formal training in economics. This category includes not only clinicians but also most NHS and DHSS administrators. Our second category is 'insider'. This refers to respondents who occupy a position within the NHS or the DHSS and who also have a background in health economics. Finally, we have used the term 'outsider' to cover respondents who are trained as economists, who are actively concerned with improving health care services, but who operate from an academic setting. The quotations from interview transcripts given below are attributed to these categories rather than to individually identified respondents.

Rationality and irrationality in the NHS

In order to understand health economists' diagnosis of the ills of the NHS and the difficulties they experience in trying to provide effective remedies, it is helpful to start by considering what they take to be rational economic action. Their basic conception of economic rationality is quite simple; that is, rational action consists in the efficient use of available means to ensure the maximum attainment of given ends. For example, in the words of an outsider, 'If behaviour is totally consistent with the objectives that the individual sets himself, I suppose that would be a quick definition of rational behaviour'. This definition is, typically couched in terms of idealized individual actors who set themselves goals and who are rational in so far as they organize their conduct in a manner that seems likely to furnish the most effective realization of those goals. However, health economists are centrally concerned not with the actions of isolated individuals but with the aggregate actions of the NHS and/or with the rational co-ordination of collective structures within the social system of health care. Consequently, the practical aim of health economics, as an applied social science, is that of establishing agreed procedures and social practices within the NHS which promote the efficient use of available means for the attainment of collective goals.

3.1

Outsider: As an economist, I would argue that efficiency matters and therefore [in relation to the NHS] it's a case of trying to build markets, institutions, etc., which support the concept of efficiency.

This characteristic formulation clearly implies that the existing structure of the NHS is relatively inefficient. This is implied because there would be no need to 'build markets and institutions' if the health care system was working reasonably well. To put this another way, it follows from the health economists' model of rational action that it is rational for them to seek to improve the running of the NHS only if their efforts and skills could not produce a better outcome elsewhere. Thus, on the assumption that health economists are behaving rationally in their own terms, the rapid growth of health economics as an applied specialism suggests that marked improvements in efficiency are possible within the NHS and that there is a reasonable likelihood of successful intervention. The ultimate objective of such intervention is to make the collective actions of the NHS resemble more closely the economists' model of the rational economic actor.

Without exception, the health economists we interviewed depicted the NHS as a singularly inefficient, and therefore irrational, organization. The main features of their portrayal were as follows. In the first place, they emphasized that the structure of the NHS is unduly weighted in favour of medical provision at the expense of administrative services. As a result, administrative departments are unable to cope properly with the flow of work and, in particular, are unable to generate the basic information without which rational administrative decisions are impossible. The following graphic account is taken from an interview with an outsider.

3.2
Outsider: The NHS is grossly under-administrated. The government proudly says they only spend 4 per cent on administration; it's just crazy, nobody knows anything about what is going on. You go down to the local hospital, we have no idea what doctors are doing, we have no idea of what the costs are of what they are doing, there is no management budgeting system. [See Ch. 6.] So there is no routine information that a firm would normally use in managing an enterprise. The chairman of the local health authority is a guy from Rowntree Mackintosh. He was absolutely appalled. He is used to knowing the price of a bag of Smarties and all this sort of thing. He rolls into this place, he has never done anything in the health service before, and is absolutely amazed that nobody knows anything. They have not got any cost data; they have not got much activity data; the planning is just in its infancy. So the NHS has a very limited capacity to do its own management and planning and they recognize that.

The underdeveloped state of NHS administration is due in large measure, it is said, to the powerful position of clinicians within the NHS. Our health economists stressed that clinicians' training diverts their attention from economic factors and creates a situation in which economic considerations are treated as marginal.

3.3
Outsider: The way in which clinicians are trained in medical

school is very much to look to the clinical effects of their interventions. They just do *not* get trained in any way at all to look at *costs*. Therefore a clinician typically makes decisions on an individual basis, without looking over his shoulder at resource consequences. There is no management system there that tells him what the resource consequences are. He usually has *no idea* how much money he is spending. It comes as a great shock to him when you begin to generate information which tells him what his costs are. Most of them are spending half a million I suppose, in terms of their consequences for nurses, beds and goodness knows what, but they have got no detailed ideas.

Health economists maintained that, as a result of the widespread lack of concern with economic consequences and of the pervasive lack of relevant information, critical decisions inevitably come to be based on *ad hoc* and often irrelevant considerations. In the following passage, an insider develops this point in the course of what she calls 'a digression on growth money'.

3.4

Insider: You have your growth money and districts bid up. . . . We have certain pools of money, and they have a label on them; and districts say, 'Can I have some of this money to do this?' Districts ask for money on the basis that they're developing a service, and they're going to see more patients, therefore they need the money. . . . So you have a whole collection of these bids, and this district's asked for £20,000, this district's asked for £50,000. And you say, we've got £1 million, how are we going to share that out? And it's just sort of finger in the wind, as to which of these bids you think – you always have far more bids than you have money. So on what basis do you allocate your resources? It's a classic resource allocation that economists are always going on about. So what happened in the past is that you had some of, 'Well, this district deserves them, we haven't given them any for a while', or, 'Well, this district they've been quite good, they did a deal with us on something else – let's reward them', or, 'Well yes, this is a really pressing need, the MP here has been kicking up a fuss'. So, there's all sorts of decision-making that's going on, which is in a sense not very rational, and also is based on costs alone.

Interviewer: Can you say what you mean by not very rational?

Insider: Well, a whole collection, the fact that one district was being rewarded, another district is because the MP's been kicking up a fuss.

The central claim being made here is that growth money, like other resources, is being allocated irrationally, that is, with no systematic appraisal of the costs and likely benefits of the various possible courses of action. Such a view was sometimes echoed by medical practitioners, as in the following quotation from a practitioner who had collaborated with health economists in a study of his own specialism.

3.5

Practitioner: Until four or five years ago, money didn't exist in the health service as far as doctors were concerned. It was almost rather like a communist state. It was quite amazing. Everybody thought what they wanted to do in their own little speciality and on the whole, provided you were patient with the system, the money tended to arrive, certainly within this hospital . . . and you could almost go out and do almost what you wanted, provided you accepted it would take one or two years for the money to actually filter through.

Interviewer: That sounds a really good thing.

Practitioner: It was, but it was dependent on an ever increasing amount of money being available. And it was also unfair in the sense that people who were prepared to shout loudest and banged the table loudest perhaps got a disproportionate share of the cash. I suppose if you talk to administrators they would say that you had a health service then that was entirely in the model of what *doctors* wanted, rather than necessarily what the community wanted. Hospital doctors are very specialized people who on the whole see life through a very narrow channel of their own speciality . . . so that they may not, almost certainly wouldn't be taking the broader view of what the community as a whole needed.

Health economists frequently stressed that NHS administrators were little better than doctors in their inability to take the 'broader view' that is required in order to make the health service contribute most effectively to the needs of the larger community. In relation to costs, for example, health economists suggested that NHS administrators tend to concentrate on internal costs expressed in financial terms instead of considering, as does the economist, every kind of cost no matter what form it takes or where it is incurred. (See the discussion of health economists and accountants in Ch. 2.) One reason for this supposed failure on the part of the health service administrators is, of course, that they lack the conceptual apparatus of the trained economist and the technical skills that would enable them to begin to assess costs in a more complete and satisfactory manner.

Our health economists maintained that this lack of suitable training is even more evident in relation to outcomes or benefits; and it is here that many of them expected in due course to be able to make a major contribution to improving the rationality of the NHS. The following outsider speaks of the dearth of information about the benefits furnished by general practitioners, but similar statements were regularly made in the interviews about various medical specialisms as well as the hospital system as a whole.

3.6

Outsider: Essentially 25 per cent of the NHS budget goes to primary care and a large lump of that primary care goes to GPs. The GPs don't have a very sensible contract. The contract says something like they have to provide the average amount of general medical care, and that is what your average GP has got to do. Nobody knows what the average GP provides. What do you know about your GP compared with my GP? There is no information available.

Our health economists argued that the lack of administrative information in the NHS, the crude and irregular estimation of costs, and the inability to measure medical outcomes or their benefits for the wider community produce a context in which political struggle provides the basic mechanism for the allocation of economic resources. In the words of the practitioner quoted above, in such an administrative situation, funds are likely to go to those who 'shout the loudest and bang the table the loudest' (3.5). It also means, of course, that the demands of well-established, prestigious medical specialisms are more likely to be satisfied. Health economists insisted that one of the major sources of inefficiency in the NHS is that the medical profession is not only exceptionally powerful but is also internally divided, so that the provision of medical services is often decided by a power struggle between groupings whose representatives hide their pursuit of vested interests behind what one outsider called 'a mumbo jumbo about clinical acceptability'. An important long-term aim of health economics is therefore to reduce the ascendancy of this self-interested 'mumbo jumbo' by the introduction of the technical discourse of economic evaluation. In the words of another outsider, economics is to be employed 'to help you crack problems of hierarchy and stagnation and inflexibility to make more effective use of resources. It's about creating a language and a cutting edge for managers'.

These are some of the major ills of the NHS that were identified in interviews by our respondents. Such a diagnosis inevitably implies the need for certain kinds of remedial action on the part of health economists. In the first place, it seems that they may be able to help by using their special 'bag of tools' to provide the missing information without which rational choices cannot be made. More specifically, health economists should be able to devise better measures of costs and benefits than are currently available within the NHS. In addition, they could perhaps provide evaluative procedures that will require practitioners to formulate their objectives more clearly and to adopt a broader view when considering alternative ways of accomplishing these objectives. In general, their goal would be to replace *ad hoc* and politically motivated decision-making, as far as possible, with an impersonal means–end calculus analogous to that characteristic of the idealized individual actor which provides their basic model of economic rationality.

The preceding paragraph should not be taken as a definitive account of the collective aims of health economics. It is, rather, our attempt, as outside observers, to provide a brief summary of the policy that seems to be implicit in their talk about the defects of the NHS and about their own efforts to improve the situation. We must stress, however, that each health economist, and each recognizable group of health economists, would formulate these aims differently in accordance with their unique position within the social world of health economics and in the light of their special skills and interests. In other words, there is no explicit, generally agreed programme for British health economics. Nevertheless, it is clear from our interviews, and is illustrated in the quotations reproduced in this chapter, that health economists are collectively committed to making the economic practices of the NHS more rational and that their concept of rationality implies the need for greater uniformity of action throughout the system, more systematic appraisal of ends and means across the full range of economic decisions, a significant reduction in the influence of political factors within the system of health care, and the widespread use of allocative procedures designed in accordance with the basic concepts of economic theory.

Insider problems

In this section we will examine some of the major problems encountered by health economists operating *within* the formal system of health care. Let us begin with a quotation from an outsider who had previously worked on the inside.

3.7

Outsider: The health service is a large but not very well understood, huge bureaucracy. It's a sort of central planning system. If we knew how it operated we might better – we might be able to release the potential that's there.

Whereas the NHS is an immense organization, the community of health economists consists of no more than a few hundred people. Thus those who choose to work on the inside are faced with a daunting problem of scale. The very size, complexity, internal diversity and widespread geographical distribution of the health care system constitutes a fundamental barrier to the success of their efforts. For, as a consequence of these features, their ability to grasp the overall structure of the system is restricted, and their influence is dispersed, swamped and negated, to a considerable degree, by the very practices which they seek to change.

The aims of the insiders, in the most general terms, are to guide the decisions in which they are directly involved towards greater rationality and to encourage the adoption by other health service personnel of more rational decision-making procedures. Health economists find themselves, however, in a context where the majority of participants have quite different primary objectives and quite different backgrounds and social allegiances. Furthermore, not only is the economists' version of rational action often unwelcome in this setting, but the very role of 'health economist' is not yet a well-established part of the bureaucratic structure. Although the following ex-insider makes this point in relation to the DHSS, it applies equally to the NHS.

3.8

Outsider: After two years I had more than enough of the DHSS, although I enjoyed it, found it very interesting, but very frustrating.

Interviewer: Why was it frustrating?

Outsider: Well principally because economists don't have a clear niche in the organization. You're an appendage that is there at the discretion of the administrative stroke medical hierarchies, which are clear hierarchies. You tend therefore to be asked for advice, although it's very much a question that it could be ignored or taken on board, but there's no sort of formal way to have any sort of comeback about being ignored. You can't argue a case. It's an advisory situation.

One consequence of insiders' marginal status, as health economists, is that their special skills are often diverted, ignored or misunderstood, and they find themselves being required to perform tasks which they regard as trivial or inappropriate.

3.9

Insider: One of the things that I found extremely typical of the practising health economist working on planning questions in the service, was that there was an enormous difference between what *I* thought economics was about and the popular perception of what economics was about; to the extent that you got shuffled into areas where you had no competence and kept out of areas where you might possibly have helped them and people were persistently trying to turn you into cost accountants.

3.10

Insider: What they need is a spare pair of hands to do some other task. If you admit that you know something about statistics . . . then they will get you doing statistics. . . . Also, if you have an economist who's on *your* team, then you can *use* him as a cost accountant because you don't trust or you don't like the cost accountants that you're normally dealing with.

In these two passages the health economists concerned speak as junior personnel whose activities are determined by the decisions of more senior staff. They thereby reveal another major difficulty likely to face any group of social scientists entering a well-established bureaucracy in a piecemeal fashion; namely, they will tend to be allowed in initially only at the lower levels, and consequently their contributions will be regulated by practitioners whose appreciation of their objectives and special skills will be quite limited. According to our respondents, both insiders and outsiders, this has certainly been the case for health economists in Britain.

3.11

Outsider: Most of these people are very junior, therefore they do not have the stripes on their arm, therefore they cannot get into high level meetings and therefore they may miss a lot of opportunities for using economics. They are treated as junior members of staff, which they *are,* which is fair enough but that really does affect their access *to* the system and their *contribution* to the system.

3.12

Insider: Unless it's done in a substantial way, my experience is that they get colonized by the largest part of the organization to which they're attached. So if they're attached to a planning department, they very quickly become colonized and become planners and there's no longer – then they lose some of the cutting edge that they came with. My impression is that often they're taken in too young, and too inexperienced, to know quite what a health economics service might be.

The conduct of insiders is, it seems, severely constrained by their location in a pre-existing hierarchical structure. They have no choice but to respond to the immediate practical demands placed upon them by medical and administrative practitioners. Our interviewees emphasized that these demands are not for long-term, economically rational solutions conceived in terms of the system as a whole, but for help in solving the pressing problems of the moment within their particular region of the bureaucratic structure. The insiders to whom we talked stressed repeatedly that, in this context, the rational perspective and the standards of technical adequacy which they had acquired in the academic world, needed considerable modification.

3.13

Insider: It does upset me sometimes that you see some *appalling* costing work going on, and if only clinicians could be put in touch with the right people at the right time then I think that would help enormously. I suppose in a lot of ways I would think that if consultants are trying to look at costs *and* benefits, then you should just encourage them, but unfortunately you often get the feeling that they're just trying to prove a case. But, no I wouldn't be too purist, because [a colleague] and I are both working on this same option appraisal [see Ch. 7] and we were actually initially given three weeks to do all the costing side. So we said, as long as we're working on the back of the same envelope then that's all that matters. And one half of me is saying all of this, and the other half of me is actually *doing literally* back-of-the-envelope calculations – for millions of pounds.

Interviewer: Do you think academic health economists would object to that when you say . . .

Insider: Yes, yes absolutely.

Interviewer: Do you think they're wrong?

Insider: This is where I get very cynical and very patronizing, but I really think that they don't know what the real world's about. They really don't know how decisions are taken in the health service, what time tables you're working to, what information you have to hand, the process. They don't understand the process that you're going through to do things. The fact that what you're just hoping for is a bigger and better envelope, it's still often the back-of-the-envelope calculation. Also you work on a *gut* feeling a lot of the time, and that only comes from experience.

Interviewer: Not very rational!

Insider: No, I know it's not very rational. I know, I, I, I (*Laugh*), well yeah, no it's not.

3.14

Insider: Most of the work that we do doesn't lift our horizons beyond the NHS and the money that is devoted to it, to the very much wider issues of what should public expenditure be doing? and the trade-offs and all of those kinds of things. And it would be, from a management point of view, foolish to go anywhere near them because you just wouldn't make decisions.

Interviewer: Because they are too big?

Insider: Because they are too far away from what you as a manager can influence.

These quotations suggest that there is a clash between, on the one hand, health economists' training, which encourages them to consider wider horizons and to undertake careful appraisal of options before making choices and, on the other hand, the narrow, pragmatic, short-term focus of those responsible for the day-to-day running of the health service. In this clash, it is clear, the health economists have to give way, to make the greater concessions. They have to stop being 'purist' and to learn to make do with economic evaluations that are inevitably 'quick and dirty' or 'back of the envelope'. These evocative phrases were employed repeatedly by our respondents to convey that, within the NHS, their attempts to implement economic rationality have to be radically simplified and put into operation over the shortest possible time span. As a result, they readily acknowledged, their actual contribution to the health care system often falls far short of their hopes and their intentions. But, they insisted, in the real world of the NHS, they have no choice but to adapt to the requirements of a system which does not favour their form of rationality.

3.15

Insider: I remember [a colleague] saying, 'Well, the trouble is', he said, 'the *last* thing the health service wants is rational decision-making'. And I think, to some extent, he'd hit the nail right on the head there.

Despite these difficulties, insiders maintained when talking to us that their efforts are by no means worthless. It is better, they said, that *some* decisions should be based on *some* information, no matter how crude, instead of on guesswork. Furthermore, they suggested, the direct involvement of health economists in particular decisions tends to encourage greater consideration of, and more open debate about, a wider range of alternatives than would otherwise be the case. In other words, insiders claim that they do help to a modest degree to widen the horizon of decision-making within the NHS, to provide some kind of factual basis for the decisions in which they are involved, and to make the procedures of decision-making more explicit and open to rational appraisal.

It is clear, however, that the provision of factual information and the systematic appraisal of alternative courses of action in no way guarantee what the health economist would regard as rational decision-making. For the conclusions of the insider are often simply ignored when, it seems, they conflict with what the health economist takes to be the interests, or the prejudices, of more powerful participants.

3.16

Insider: About two years ago we did a load of analysis . . . for our district. And it went in front of the district administrators. And it didn't tell them what they wanted to know, it told them the exact opposite. . . . Loads and loads of work done on it, huge report, loads of detail, and [they] just said 'data's wrong' and that was it, the data is wrong. Therefore what we then had to do was go through a huge three-month exercise tidying up the data in conjunction with the districts. And it was really just a ploy, 'Get these people off our backs, get them to do something else'. If we'd gone along with that report and it had shown the opposite, not *one* of them would have questioned the data, they wouldn't have said, 'We can't believe this, we know your data's rubbish'. They just would have said, 'Oh yes, damn fine report that, and thank you very much'.

On other occasions, it appears, the 'facts' and/or the 'rational procedures' furnished by the health economist may meet with a more positive response because they can be used as part of the rhetoric of persuasion in a decision-making process that is essentially political. In the following passage, an insider describes how this political context has sometimes directly influenced his use of the language and techniques of economics.

3.17

Insider: I suppose if I am honest I've on occasion provided some very useful economic arguments to back up a decision that has already been made by whoever wants it to be made in order to get it through the necessary bits of political machinery. . . . It's like anything else; we can't preserve our purity. . . . I think it is a natural limitation of anything in a real-world setting where there are real, difficult decisions to be made. There are power relationships and all of those kinds of things. In that kind of situation you use any of the weapons you have available to you, and if spurious rationality is helpful, why not use it?

Interviewer: Does measurement or quantification have a particular power in these practical negotiations?

Insider: Oh yes. It has enormous power. Oh yes.

Interviewer: Who is impressed by it? I mean any particular set of actors more than others?

Insider: Yes, the least knowledgeable. I mean, we have done very well in the regional capital programme because we have been very studious in producing very kosher option appraisals for all our capital proposals. . . . And I am sure we have got more things more quickly than we would have done if we had just been like all the other districts. Now the quality of the economics in any or all of that is poor to non-existent, but the structure and the framework of economics makes it all look very good. Maybe I am being overcritical of ourselves there, because sometimes we have surprised ourselves: we have done appraisals and we've actually come to a conclusion that we thought we weren't going to come to, and we have made better decisions as a result. But not always. On some occasions there have been political factors, which perhaps is difficult to talk about, in the arena where the decisions have to be made, or objectives that have never been stated but have been implicitly there.

As this quotation illustrates, a pervasive underlying problem for economists who work on the *inside* is that, in entering the system, they inevitably sacrifice their autonomy. As members of the health care bureaucracy, their primary obligations are to other members of that bureaucracy rather than to the academic economists from whom they learnt their skills and from whom they acquired their conception of economic rationality. It is because they are insiders that they are subordinate to non-economists, immersed in practical day-to-day affairs and caught up in the politics of the NHS. It may be, therefore, that by remaining on the outside health economists can retain greater autonomy and avoid some of these difficulties. In the next section, we will consider the pros and cons of attempting to intervene in the operation of the health service from a distance.

The pros and cons of working on the outside

It follows from the discussion in the previous section that one of the main benefits for health economists of being located outside the health care system is that of autonomy. Outsiders regularly maintained in the interviews that their independence of the formal bureaucratic structure enables them to be more impartial in considering its problems, to be more openly critical of its defects and also to spend more time exploring possible solutions that require long-term investigation.

3.18

Outsider: Some people who understand enough about economics believe that it introduces a greater amount of objectivity. Now whether that is justified or not I am not sure. If for example I was working as an economist *in* the health service, I think life would be more difficult for me. One has a certain freedom as an academic, but one can also be a bit more detached in being not part of the organization and therefore one can be critical. And I think given the stance of an *academic* health economist one can perhaps be relatively objective and value-free in terms of health care policies – besides these underlying value-judgements of equity and efficiency. If you take some of the studies we have been involved in, acting as consultants to the NHS, such as the closure of beds in a London district, I honestly didn't care which beds were closed; whether it was this hospital or that hospital *except* in terms of efficiency and equity. . . . Some of the work that I have done . . . is pretty far away from being capable of being applied as it stands. I think it is the idea of fundamental research as opposed to applied research. Very often research, if it *is* going to have policy relevance or it *is* going to have practical application, it will be some years before it is worked up to that level. Health status measurement, for example, for a long time was really largely at a level of conceptual and theoretical work. It is only more recently it has got to being applied.

Some outsiders proposed, in addition, that when they became involved in studying and in trying to change the practices of the NHS, they have the advantage of not being allied with any internal faction and that they are therefore more likely to elicit honest responses from practitioners on which to base their practical recommendations.

3.19

Outsider: The problem with being an insider, I think, is that people are less willing to go along with you and, if you like, be *honest* about their own values, their own judgements about fact. Because then you'll probably be identified with a group, a faction, within the organization and that may make it harder to be effective. So it has some disadvantages as well. For some kind of problems it's better to be an insider. I mean if you've got things where there isn't a lot of conflict around; where there *is* a problem, there's perceived to be a problem, but there's not a lot of conflict, you haven't got warring factions, then it's probably better to be an insider. Where you've got major conflict between groups, it's probably better to have an outsider coming in.

The previous speaker proposed that insiders have the great advantage of knowing their 'local patch' intimately and that, as long as the issues in question are not particularly contentious, this advantage will often enable them to apply their economic skills more effectively than outsiders of similar experience. However, when there is division within the NHS, he suggested, the non-aligned outsider is much more likely to be successful because his conclusions will be free from the taint of sectional interest. Outsiders regularly maintained that the nature of their intellectual community, their academic concerns and their location outside the health care system, made them almost entirely immune from political influences.

3.20

Outsider: Although I work closely with [certain other health economists] they are not telling me what to think in the same way as, or sending me signals about what to think in the same way as, say, an undersecretary of the British Medical Association has to think a certain way. In the BMA, the thinking is dominated by the interests of the collectivity. . . . Well what keeps me in the academic life, I think above all, is some sense of freedom, in the sense that I feel that although undersecretaries or high officials of organizations may be more powerful, they are ultimately serfs; while we are ultimately free men, in the sense that we can take initiatives, and we do. They may be in quite small spheres, but they do represent a sort of free play of mind, to a greater extent than, say, civil servants in the DHSS.

3.21

Interviewer: When you get into the area of incentives aren't you becoming a totally political actor?

Outsider: No, I don't think so. I mean what you are trying to do is ask the question, where you have got some sets of incentives now, you have got some alternative sets of incentives, and the interesting question intellectually is what are the relative effects of those two sets of incentives. So the thing that *I'm* going to be arguing is incentives – changing incentives is part of a political game, you might argue. As an *academic* what I am interested in is emphasizing that we don't know what the effects of these incentives are and must experiment in careful trials. . . . So that is the thrust of the academic bit.

Outsiders repeatedly claimed that their independence enables them to gather accurate information about the operation of the NHS, to use this information as the basis for advice which is seen to be disinterested, and therefore to help resolve differences of opinion inside the health care bureaucracy and to propel the NHS towards greater efficiency. Clearly, this kind of account implies that the relevant parties within the NHS are capable of accepting and acting upon the advice received from outsiders. In the following passage, an insider suggests that there is a rational mechanism at work which encourages implementation, namely, that payment for specific external consultancies encourages careful assessment of the economic benefits that may ensue.

3.22

Insider: Continually you're thinking: Nice bloke, but £350 a day, or £200 or £100 or whatever the price is – Now is it worth it? What else could I be buying with those funds? . . . So there is that continual test.

This speaker suggested that, in order to receive regular commissions, outsiders have to establish a reputation for providing useful results. If their advice fails to pay off, they will quickly be eliminated from the consultancy market. This view seems to assume that the recipients of outsiders' recommendations will be in reasonable agreement about the nature of the initial problem and about the effectiveness of the health economists' proposals. As we have seen, however, in many cases outsiders will be consulted precisely because internal agreement is lacking. In such circumstances, the formal provision of data and advice is not enough; outsiders have to enter into direct discussion with practitioners and use their special skills to encourage them to adopt the same cool, detached perspective as their external consultants.

3.23

Outsider: The tools and framework of cost–benefit analysis have been applied *extremely* successfully in my experience . . . in resolving conflict and getting people to come to agreed decisions in areas where previously they were unable to reach decisions. I think the subject has offered a framework within which people could actually come to an understanding of how they were trading-off various choices, and therefore could achieve a consensus view on how it *should* be done. First of all, I think the technique helps with actually thinking clearly about options themselves, about choices you *could* make . . . it helps in the structuring of the problem; it helps in getting them to generate alternatives for solving the problem; and then when you've got alternatives, some of which are good on some dimensions and bad on others, and some of them are reversed, how you can cope with the fact you're having to make trade-offs then. So it helps them to go through the process of actually identifying what the trade-offs are, and then coming to a view about whether or not they want to make one trade-off rather than another. . . . And in my experience it's very rare for the people involved to renege on the, or *try* to renege on the process, whereby, having got the result which they didn't want out of it, they'll say, 'Alright, well, I'm willing to accept that because I've been involved in the process by which that decision was made, and at each individual step it looked right'.

The more well-known outsiders, like the speaker in 3.23, have access to many different parts of the health care system. As a result, they can apply their knowledge when and where it is needed and they can ensure that new ideas and techniques are quickly disseminated. Whereas internal expertise is relatively immobile and its results organizationally confined, that of the outsider can be made to work for the benefit of the NHS as a whole. This idea is put forward in the following illustrative passage, where the respondent begins by referring to the work of the speaker in 3.23.

3.24

Outsider: He has been the catalyst in producing a structure which is saleable and acceptable to the end users who *don't* want to reinvent the wheel, who *do* want something which is productive in terms of their time, has a definable outcome which they – they are not going to take on any risks in adopting this evaluative procedure themselves because they know it has worked in other settings. So they know it's got a good track record and he has helped in that learning process because he has made mistakes for other people. He is coming up with a clean product in which they can be pretty well assured that they are not going to make the same mistakes as he has.

Interviewer: So that kind of thing can be transferrable to completely different contexts?

Outsider: Yes. I mean that sort of experience undertaken by, or achieved by, people working outside of the health service or in collaboration with the health service or perhaps funded to do the work in an academic environment using the health authority as a test bed, I think is an extremely useful approach and one which I think ought to be increasingly adopted to ensure the maximum gain for everybody; because I don't think health authorities always have the resources to say to other health authorities, 'Look this is what we have been about and it worked and it's great and why don't you try it'. Whereas if a university encapsulates that experience in working collaboratively with a health authority, they are not going to sit on their hands, they are going to be saying to the world: 'This is, if not *the* way, certainly a very useful way of going forward'.

This outsider, like the others quoted so far in this section, offers a strongly positive image of direct intervention from outside the system, an image which is reminiscent of the strong programme discussed in the preceding chapter. The picture we are given in these passages is that of an independent intellectual community whose members are free to use the basic principles of economic theory to devise rational techniques relevant to the practical problems of the NHS and are able, on the whole, to put these techniques into practice in a manner which surmounts the hierarchical barriers and political antagonisms that undermine and distort the efforts of their colleagues inside the system. However, this is undoubtedly an idealized representation which outsiders themselves seldom furnished without qualification. They mentioned, for example, that their autonomy is inevitably limited in practice and that they, like insiders, but to a lesser degree, are subject to the pressure for 'quick and dirty' results. Insiders expressed stronger reservations about the benefits of working on the outside and were likely to insist that outsiders often have a mistaken and inflated idea of their effectiveness in the real world of the NHS (see, for example, 3.13). Let us look in a little more detail at what our respondents, both insiders and outsiders, had to say about the problems of intervention from the outside.

Insiders, in their accounts of these problems, repeatedly emphasized that the academic economics community has its own intellectual momentum which prevents its members from responding adequately to the needs of the health care service. In the following quotation, an insider is commenting on what he takes to be the unduly academic focus of the Health Economists' Study Group, which provides the main forum for debate among British health economists.

3.25

Insider: They seemed to be more concerned with econometric aspects [which] didn't seem to me particularly practically related to the decisions that need to be made on a day-to-day basis – even as a regional health authority – for planning and development. Of course it's a very catholic group, and there are many there who wouldn't see econometrics as being the central core of the field of interests of the people in that group. I suppose I just got fed up. But I think it was symptomatic of a real problem they have with their group: that if it's going to have influence within the NHS, then it does need to keep an ear to what practitioners in the field – whether they're from finance departments, or whether they're from planning departments, whether they're from administration or medicine – are saying to them. What I was trying to say to them was: 'I don't have confidence that what you're talking about is relevant to the kinds of things I see in front of me'.

Respondents employed within the health care bureaucracy maintained that usually what was needed from outsiders, as from insiders, was direct practical help in solving practitioners' immediate difficulties. They insisted that the NHS was not asking outsiders for rational techniques or for a special way of thinking, but merely for assistance in achieving their goals in a situation where internal administrative resources are insufficient.

3.26

Insider: What the customer is looking for is usually what he considers to be comparatively *modest* help, and work which the organization would quite well be able to do if it could just delegate somebody who was already in the organization. There's quite enough ideas and clear thinking. What is especially being offered [by the health economist] is gathering those ideas together in a more concrete framework than they previously had been, and estimating the values to put upon various of those ideas and doing some quantification. So it's a combination of quantification and the clearer statement of ideas that are already around. I think there are very few people in the health service who would slap their thighs and say, 'Ah! We need some clear thinking, call in the health economist'. . . . I think that's what he *thinks* he's offering, and would like to be offering, but I don't think he's going to get many contracts if he puts in his prospectus, 'What I can offer you is clearer thinking than you've ever had before'.

It seems, from repeated statements of this kind, that outside health economists are likely to interpret their contribution to, and their relationship with, the NHS rather differently from those working within the system. From the point of view of the latter, constant efforts have to be made to prevent outsiders from doing too much, too late and from too academic a perspective.

3.27

Insider: We've got the problem of fitting into *their* programme and getting a response, which can take a little while to get that response. And when we get it, the work tends to be perhaps better done, but more thoroughly done, than we actually need. . . . They will insist that it's done as a proper academic study and rightly in an academic [unclear], but that isn't what we're actually looking for.

For outsiders, of course, this is the recurrent problem of being forced by pressure of circumstance to carry out 'quick and dirty' studies instead of the careful, rigorous investigations which are, in their view, essential if significant, lasting improvements in the economics of health care are to be achieved. Despite their relative autonomy, outsiders tend to portray themselves as constantly adapting to the everyday requirements of the health care system and, like insiders, as adjusting their academic standards accordingly.

3.28

Outsider: The managers want instant information to make decisions now . . . that is why we made this very deliberate decision to create this [new unit]. Because what we want to do is differentiate between really two types of activity. So that the [new unit] is going to be much more a management consultancy, 'quick and dirty' as we use the phrase, back of the envelope and off you go lads, give 'em an answer tomorrow. That is what they are going to be wanting: quick – and they are accepting it's dirty – analysis. They want somebody to sweep in there, collect lots of numbers, grind it all up and tell them what the numbers, the tea leaves, tell them what happens.

Interviewer: But if there is no credence to the numbers, what do they want that stuff for?

Outsider: Well the argument crudely would be that some information is better than none and they haven't any at the moment. So if you sweep in there and concentrate your and their minds on it for six months and collect the data that *can* be collected in that period, sort of put it into some sort of framework and give it to them, fair enough. But I think the other thing which is very important is that the [new unit] is going to be very much a mechanism for identifying *areas* where you can do research. So if you like the [new unit] can sort of sweep over a field and drop out a few things and then the old researchers can sort of trot along later on.

In this passage, the speaker suggests that he and his colleagues have begun to develop a strategy which separates short-term practical projects from more thorough, academically defined studies. In this way, it is implied, they can satisfy the practical demands of the NHS without sacrificing their academic integrity and without abandoning the ultimate goal of trying to provide the analytical basis for radical change in health care practice. How outsiders respond to this dilemma is likely to depend on the particular kind of group in which they operate and on the nature of their funding. In the next passage, another outsider comments on the same problem. Like all our respondents, whether outsiders or insiders, his view is that, whatever else they do, health economists have no choice but to meet the immediate requirements of their customers.

3.29

Outsider: There has been a lot of discussion about should we produce studies, more timely studies, that are less well done, just to knock things in the right direction rather than trying to come up with a definitive study after the decision has been made; and so there's a pressure for quick and dirty studies. At the time I was at York, the word was that we were slow and dirty [*Laughter*]. But I think there is some sort of trade-off, I mean it's part of the game I suppose of trying to be policy-relevant, isn't it? . . . I think whether or not you feel it's important in terms of credibility, would depend where you came from. If you were formerly a mainstream economist, or worked in a place like York which has its links with the Economics Department, you'd probably be worried about that because you'd be continually being subjected to your peers' criticisms. If you're in another setting like mine, or in a medical school, you'd probably be less worried about it. But I think it's just a problem that we have to face. . . . I mean adequacy must be adequacy to the particular context, appropriate and adequate to the decision that has to be made. And if a decision has to be made in six months, then something that takes nine months is inadequate. . . . It's difficult to be detailed, thorough, comprehensive, quickly. Now, to the extent that those three are often seen as academic virtues, then it's difficult to be thoroughly respectable academically, quickly. But, in a sense, so what?

Outsiders persistently represent themselves, like the speaker in 3.29, as departing radically from academic standards and objectives in much of their work in order to ensure that their efforts are useful in concrete terms. Participants *within* the health care system, however, as we have noted (3.25–7), are nevertheless inclined to criticize them for being too academic and for failing to meet their practical needs in full. It seems that, whilst the health economists' long-term aim is to reform the NHS according to the requirements of their model of rational action, the representatives of the NHS are striving to employ the economists' expertise for their own very different, internally defined ends. Neither party is entirely satisfied with the resulting compromise. But it seems that the NHS is the more powerful protagonist in this struggle over the correct way to deploy the health economists' bag of tools and that even those economists who operate from outside the system are continually forced to make concessions and to modify or to defer their more ambitious aspirations. We saw earlier that outsiders sometimes argue that there is an economic mechanism which promotes the implementation of their recommendations (3.22). However, it can also be argued that there is an even more pervasive economic mechanism which enables those who provide the funds largely to determine what sorts of studies are undertaken in the first place.

3.30

Interviewer: Would you say there's been a direct influence of particular patterns of funding on the growth or the pattern of growth of health economics?

Outsider: Yeah, I would say it's been enormous. You can only explain half the things we research in terms of the funder's interest. . . . A lot of it could be useful but it's not particularly independent. I'm not knocking it, but the fact of the matter is that the DHSS says it wants a particular area studied: say the impact of joint funding. Now in this day I wouldn't think many independent scholars would sit down and say that was one of the human race's most important problems [*Laugh*]. I mean it's the sort of minor logging of bureaucratic tramp steamers over their sea routes.

Interviewer: That does sound as if you're knocking it actually. That sounds as if you're saying that there's a lot of duff work gets done because somebody wants it done, and people are prepared to do it for no reason other than the fact that somebody's paying for it.

Outsider: Well, I am saying there's a danger that there could be very important topics that get neglected because people won't really pay for them.

3.31

Outsider: Ideally one would like funding that is absolutely neutral. But tell me what funding is absolutely neutral? The DHSS funding, it seems to me, really has many problems. Funding by anyone who's got an interest in the results you come up with and may prefer you to come up with one answer rather than another, for some reason of their own, has got its problems.

It seems, in the light of various statements along these lines, that the formal autonomy of many outsiders is less significant than their financial dependence on the health care bureaucracy. This dependence is particularly evident in the case of younger researchers who are not part of any clearly defined career structure and who are able to maintain a regular income only by accepting a series of short-term contracts. In such circumstances, outsiders maintained, they have no choice but to take whatever job is on offer and to move quickly from one topic to another in accordance with the requirements of the commissioning agencies. Furthermore, like insiders in comparably minor positions, they seem to find that the internal structure of the NHS creates major difficulties for them as they attempt to pursue their research and, in the interviews, they tended to express dissatisfaction with the adequacy of their own work and with that of others trying to investigate the NHS from the outside. The speaker in the following passage touches on several of these issues.

3.32

Outsider: I think you have got to distinguish between the individuals here who are soft-money funded, and there are a lot of them having fixed-term contracts with grants that don't roll over, as part of a programme with a termination date – and junior researchers who have just come into research maybe as a result of doing the [degree] programme or being recruited as a body into a research programme because they are affordable. Individuals like that . . . expect to do three years of dog's-body type of research for other people before they gain a little bit of academic respectability having got three or four papers on their CV and then that gives them a chance to apply for something more exotic. I think there are others who take their research very seriously because possibly they can afford to do so either because there is more security in the sense of tenure, perhaps a core post [here] funded at least for, say, five years with the possibility of roll-over, where individuals have more thinking time. Whereas the majority of us who are on soft money have pressures of doing one research programme, looking round for other research work or other work of any sort possibly, and need to retain some sort of academic standard in terms of the quality of work you produce, which is not always easy if you are working to poor-quality research design or with or for researchers who have little grasp of the subject.

Interviewer: You have no control of how the research goes?

Outsider: Yes, I mean any protocol doesn't hold up nine times out of ten, and certainly if you are expected to work in the health service or with the health service you're very largely dependent upon your ability to persuade the establishment of the viability and scientific *type* of what you propose doing, the chances of there being a successful outcome, the need for minimal inputs from their end. And all the time there are competing demands in terms of actually realizing the protocol. . . . From my point of view, the way forward is not to assume that anything in a hospital is possible; to assume in fact that the majority of what you want to do will create difficulties.

It is clear from interview transcripts such as that quoted in 3.32 that although outsiders' investigations are normally commissioned by or financially supported by the health care bureaucracy, this does not guarantee co-operation from the practitioners under study, nor does it necessarily enable the researchers to cope with the practical problems that inevitably arise in the course of research within the NHS. As with insiders, outsiders' relationship with the medical hierarchy appears to be critical.

3.33
Outsider: These problems mitigate against using a District General Hospital as a good test bed for research *unless* it is a top-down initiative, unless you have got these consultants saying, 'By Christ, it's absolutely imperative that we do that; I will talk to my medical team and they will be instructed from day one'.

It seems that outsiders, like insiders, are often frustrated by having to carry out their studies within a complex, hierarchical structure whose members are fully engaged, not in the search for economic rationality, but in pursuing concrete, daily objectives that are organizationally and professionally defined. Thus, despite the fact that their research projects frequently originate within the bureaucracy, outsiders experience great difficulty in producing the kind of results that are required by the commissioning agencies within the time-scale deemed to be appropriate. Nevertheless, the great majority of outsiders undoubtedly strive conscientiously to overcome these problems and to provide information – albeit quick and dirty information – that can be used to recommend changes in practice inside the NHS. Insiders tended to suggest, however, that it is at this stage that outside consultancy reveals its greatest weaknesses; namely, that the economists responsible for the recommendations have little or no say in their practical implementation and that political influences once again become crucially important.

3.34
Interviewer: So the result of an option appraisal, or other kinds of economic evaluation, if you're satisfied with how it's been done – you'd tend to implement it like that? There wouldn't be any grounds at that point for re-evaluating it?
Insider: Oh well there may be, yes, because, there may be political issues which, it was decided, wouldn't be given any weight, which turn out to be decisive. Or you may have decided just because of the flow of capital money, that you're not actually going to go ahead with the project which you evaluated, whether it was going to be in location A, location B or location C. And the whole thing is delayed. Or some other extraneous factor comes in and complicates the picture in a way which

wasn't taken account of. Oh yes, I mean there are plenty of reasons why things aren't implemented.

Interviewer: Would those reasons be deficiencies of the original study? Should they have been taken into account in the study?

Insider: Well *no*, no. You may decide quite explicitly not to take into account certain political issues. You may decide that for reasons of economy you can't do the full social investigations that you might have wanted, and so you feel a little bit uneasy about the numbers that have come out on that aspect. And if the overall magnitude of difference is between A and B you may argue, and it may be the subject of political debate as to whether a particular aspect has got sufficient attention. And then sometimes there are more complicated aspects, which for simplicity's sake, for the study you excluded, and then, in the political debate come back in. So it isn't at all straightforward.

Passages such as this strongly suggest that outsiders' findings and recommendations do not remove political negotiation from the process of decision-making; that, in many cases, outside consultancy merely defers or redirects what economists describe as 'political' factors. In fact, our interview material indicates that, because outsiders' conclusions are so frequently 'quick and dirty' or 'back of the envelope', they can often be challenged and that they become but one inconclusive element in a complex decision-making process. It seems to follow from these observations that although outsiders themselves may be largely removed from direct involvement in the politics of the NHS, this is not true of their findings, recommendations or practical proposals. How these are interpreted and put into practice seems to depend heavily on the political interests of their advocates within the NHS. It is true that outsiders do have greater formal autonomy than insiders and that this does allow them greater freedom of action. At the same time, however, it removes any possibility of their creating a power base within the system of health care from which to reconstruct its economic activities.

The formal autonomy of outsiders, which severely restricts their ability to intervene directly in the operation of the health care system, does not ensure that they are independent of that system. For as we noted earlier, outsiders cannot exist without support from the health care bureaucracy; yet this support is forthcoming only if outsiders provide results that are deemed to be valuable by members of a structure which the outsiders regard as strikingly irrational. Many of our respondents, both insiders and outsiders, recognized that, as a result of this asymmetrical relationship, the frame of reference within which outsiders undertake much of their work is set by their clients. This is partly because the health care system will only commission certain sorts of study (see 3.30), but also because health economists themselves are not inclined to pursue topics where there seems little likelihood of their research having any practical effect.

3.35

Outsider: Not a lot of work is done on systems. Not a lot of work is done in that *area* of looking at the whole of the NHS . . .

Interviewer: If the macro stuff is not being done, could you just say because nobody is commissioning you to do it?

Outsider: It's partly that but also it's partly – you know one is not totally subject to being commissioned to do things. There is a considerable amount of scope to pursue the little fancies of one's mind. And I guess it is much more exciting to do the sort of QALYs [quality adjusted life years], incentives, competition stuff, than it has been to look at the systems. Why? Because the typical response to anything to do with systems is, 'Well that's that!' You aggregate the budget of England, Scotland, Wales and Northern Ireland and you apply the RAWP [Regional Allocation Working Party] formula. You show that if you equalize the budget you reduce the Scottish budget by 17 per cent. No one is going to do anything about it. So we're back to the politics.

This, and many other similar passages in the interviews, suggest that outsiders do have some say in defining their research projects. But they also indicate that outsiders' focus of attention is greatly influenced by practitioners' concrete requirements and by what are taken to be the political realities of the situation. Some outsiders may be more able than any insiders to set the terms of their involvement with the health care system. But the supposed advantages of formal autonomy have become increasingly doubtful as we have examined the full range of respondents' comments on the nature of external consultancy. The idealized account with which this section began has been modified beyond recognition by participants themselves. As an alternative to the image of an independent intellectual community firmly guiding the NHS towards greater economic rationality, we have been shown a picture of economically dependent technical workers providing practical assistance on a commission basis for an administratively ineffective state bureaucracy. If we take this alternative picture to be less idealized and more accurate, we are led to conclude that health economists, both insiders and outsiders, in attempting to make the health care system more rational, have become caught up in, and to a large extent defeated by, the very irrationalities they set out to overcome.

However, this could be regarded as an unduly negative and unnecessarily pessimistic conclusion. Health economists might well reply that the reality is somewhere between the two extreme representations offered above and they might identify a whole series of particular studies and techniques which, despite the difficulties described in this chapter, have been successful in the sense that they have increased the level of rationality within the system of health care (see 3.23, for example). We will examine the character and effectiveness of some of the major techniques in later chapters. Let us conclude this chapter by briefly assessing health economists' own appraisals of the overall success of their enterprise so far. This will help us to decide which of the two images, if either, is the more appropriate.

Judgements of success and failure

The three following quotations reflect the general tone of health economists' evaluations, in the interviews, of the success of their collective endeavours.

3.36

Insider: I think there have been some fairly subtle changes in the practice of many clinicians and in the nature of publications as well. I am not sure economists as such have all that much credit to take for that actually, I think it is more general cultural change, the change of the whole climate in the service that has brought these things more to the fore and the rather more crude approaches to economics, of cost cutting and all the rest of it, that people are far *more* aware of than the work of economists.

3.37

Insider: One of the problems I think is that it's assumed that the language of economics and the numbers which emerge are going to be critical in bringing about reforms of attitude and behaviour; and denying by implication that there might be other more effective strategies. But I don't think the track record of health economics has been particularly promising. This is one of the things which *I* find dispiriting; there's ten years of investment of, I suppose, up to about 200 people now working in this country in health economics; all keen on reform and influencing decision-making strategy and tactics particularly within the health service. And, I don't know, it doesn't seem to have made a *fat* lot of difference.

Interviewer: So you wouldn't agree with some health economists who claim that it's very early days yet?

Insider: Oh yes it is early days yet, yes, I guess by 2000, the year 2500, we will have a clearer picture.

3.38

Outsider: It's very difficult to influence the structure of the organization from outside. And there are so few economists inside, let alone at senior levels, that we just haven't managed to cope with that at all. . . . Patience is needed. It's a bit like the Chinese water torture, drip, drip, drip, before you actually get through. But in the shorter term, actually trying to get the structures more sensible, well I despair.

These typical quotations from participants end on a note of despair. Health economists themselves, it seems, when they come to reflect informally on the progress they have made during ten years or so of concerted effort, are strongly inclined towards pessimism. They recognize that, although there have been many minor successes, they have thus far failed to make a major impact on the irrational practices that appear to them to be endemic within the health care service. But it is also evident from these quotations that, despite all the difficulties, they have not given up. Instead, in recent years, health economists have increasingly adopted a third strategy, in addition to re-education of practitioners and direct intervention in the health service, namely, that of fostering change in the NHS by entering into public debate with doctors and with other interested parties.

3.39

Outsider: I'm a believer in the clash of ideas and debate and argument. . . . What happens in this field is that there's maybe a working synthesis which survives for months or a year or two, before being overtaken by events. And then there's a new period of questioning and argument and a new synthesis. We're contributing really to this battle of ideas, though there are strong pressures in a highly bureaucratized, organized, interest-group-dominated society towards stereotyping and uniformity of thought.

Clearly, health economists intend to participate in public debate as opponents of bureaucratic inertia, factional interest and uniformity of thought. Their aim, presumably, is to employ the market-place of ideas to demonstrate to the wider community that the intellectual resources of economics can be, and should be, put to use for the medical benefit of the members of that community and, thereby, to bring pressure to bear for the implementation of more rational health care policies. Let us observe how they fare in this debate.

4 'Fury over prof's kidney call': health economists in the media

Introduction

Whilst we were carrying out the research for this book, there was much public discussion of the future of the NHS. As a result, health economists appeared regularly in the local and national media of mass communication. Their involvement reached a crescendo in 1987 with three peak-hour television programmes devoted to consideration of the QALY (quality adjusted life year): a technique for outcome measurement and resource allocation which we examine in detail in Chapter 5. As our project developed, we became increasingly aware of the public face of health economics. Scarcely a week went by without colleagues, friends or family drawing our attention to the latest pronouncements of the health economists in the media.

In this chapter we try to convey a sense of what happens when health economists enter the world of mass communication. We show how their discourse is altered, fragmented and, from their own perspective, often distorted, as it is taken over, assessed and disseminated by the numerous conflicting voices of television and the press. This semantic transformation of health economics is brought about in four ways. First, health economists themselves tend to change their style when they are put in touch with a mass audience. Second, health economists' claims and recommendations are restated, and at the same time reformulated, by the practitioners of the media. Third, the interpretative context is widened and diversified as health economists' views are placed alongside those of other interested, and usually critical, parties. Fourth, the public debate about the economics of the NHS is undertaken within the constraints imposed by textual formats designed to capture the attention of a large-scale audience and to present issues of public policy in an easily-digestible manner.

What follows in the rest of this chapter is not a conventional textual analysis but an attempt by us to re-present to the reader certain aspects of the public debate concerning health economics and its practical relevance. We have tried to recreate the style and part of the substance of that debate by reprocessing some of its textual components in accordance with the typographical practices of present day British journalism. Our treatment of the data is meant to be roughly analogous to the way in which the press selected, reorganized and dramatized *their* material on health economics and its practical policies. Thus the major part of the chapter consists of an arrangement of newspaper clippings and selections from the transcripts of television and radio programmes from the period 1985 to 1987. This material focuses on three main topics, namely, QALYs, the reform of general practitioner services, and NHS funding.

Because the health economists at York have been particularly active in the media, we obtained much of this material from the press-clipping service of the University of York. The original source for each item is given, and we have been scrupulous in retaining every error to be found in the data. Readers are advised, therefore, to examine these textual fragments with care. They are also invited to reflect on the character of the public debate mirrored in the pages below and to consider how far it is likely to increase the pressure for greater 'economic rationality' in the health service.

The chapter ends with our version of a journalistic report about this book. In this section, we have chosen to exercise the right claimed by all contributors to the media of adding our own fiction to the existing interpretative chaos.

WHO'S RIGHT, WHO'S WRONG, AND WHO DECIDES?

York's centre for health economics has recently acquired a certain notoriety. Are researchers there playing God or solving mysteries of NHS cost effectiveness?

THES (Times Higher Education Supplement) 27 Feb 87

WE all realise that today we live in a world dominated by accountants and that "cost effectiveness" is almost holy writ.

YE Post (Yorkshire Evening Post) 4 Sept 86

Professors Alan Williams and Alan Maynard seem to be operating by appointment to God.

HSJ (Health Service Journal) 9 Oct 86

Planners were urged to "get religion" and fight for community care by Nick Bosanquet of the Centre for Health Economics at the University of York.

Community Care 31 Oct 86

"Prof. Williams's formula did not drop out of heaven with a heavenly affidavit."

Yorkshire Post 3 Sept 86

Our reporters investigate

Buying health and efficiency

THES 27 Feb 87

The centre's guiding principle is to apply economic concepts and techniques to health care. It sounds a rather dull raison d'etre.

THES 27 Feb 87

Maynard: If you want to talk about value for money and efficiency you must ask how much you are spending and what you're getting out of it in terms of improved health.

'Today' BBC Radio 4, 15 Dec 87

Williams: There are now so many beneficial things that the health care system can do for people that no country . . . can afford to do them all. So we have to . . . decide what are the things that we will do and what are the things that we can't really afford to do.

'Medicine Now' BBC Radio 4, 11 Dec 86

In pursuit of performance

Hospital Equipment and Supplies Dec 86

The university began work in health economics almost 20 years ago, as an offshoot to its economics department. Since then the centre has grown to be the biggest in its field in the country. (Nearest rivals are Brunel and Aberdeen.)

Since 1983 it has been a designated research centre of the Economic and Social Research Council, funded with about £350,000 mainly from the ESRC, the Department of Health and Social Security, and privately commissioned research.

Now more than 40 staff work there on over 20 current research projects.

THES 27 Feb 87

The work by Professors Alan Williams and Alan Maynard and others deserves serious attention.

HSJ 20 Nov 86

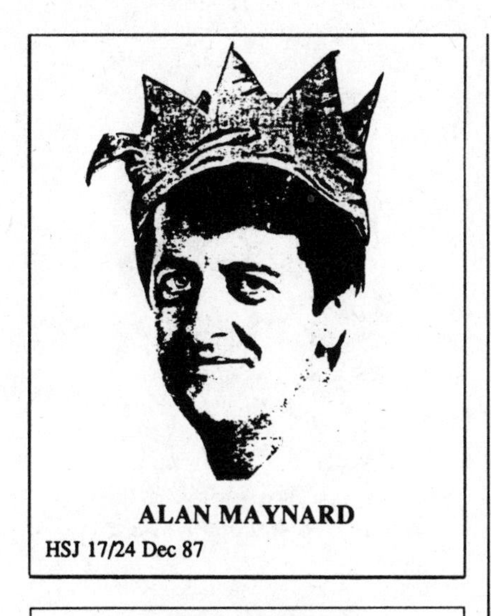

ALAN MAYNARD

HSJ 17/24 Dec 87

Who is Alan Maynard?

Professor Alan Maynard, director of the centre for health economics at York University.

Guardian 15 July 86

. . . director of the Centre for Health Education at the University of York.

Times 21 Dec 87

. . . leading health economist,

Guardian 18 June 86

. . . of the Chair of Economies at York University.

Glasgow Herald 4 Nov 87

A leading academic.

Pulse 12 Dec 87

. . . an expert in a social science.

HSJ 23 Jan 86

A professor in a blue suit with blue eyes.

Observer 12 Oct 86

Professor Alan Maynard of York University has been making rather a lot of appearances on the goggle box recently. But we had no idea that he was also becoming a pin up.

HSJ 20 Feb 87

-the man who has become the scourge of GPs.

General Practitioner 17 Oct 86

Can this be the same Professor Maynard who attacked Social Services Secretary Norman Fowler about changes in primary healthcare and who Dr Michael Wilson of the BMA referred to as a trendy academic?

HSJ 30 Jan 87

Dr Michael Wilson said: "Prof Maynard seems to go around the country peddling his idiosyncratic views."

YE Press (Yorkshire Evening Press) 4 Sept 86

Who is Alan Williams?

An economist, Prof. Alan Williams of York University.

YE Press 4 Sept 86

. . . the history professor at York University.

Doctor 9 Oct 86

A HEALTH boffin.

Northern Echo 3 Sept 86

. . . a leading economist.

Guardian 3 Sept 86

QALY-Wallies like Prof. Alan Williams and his associates at York University.

Doctor 28 May 87

Who are the others?

. . . economist Nick Bosanquet, senior research fellow at the centre for health economics at the University of York.

HSJ 23 Oct 86

. . . a Yorkshire expert.

Hull Daily Mail 20 June 86

. . . a famous health economist.

HSJ 4 June 87

Mr Bosanquet has been rather unkindly referred to as "Mr 2 per cent", following a series of exchanges between himself and former health minister Barney Hayhoe.

HSJ 23 Oct 86

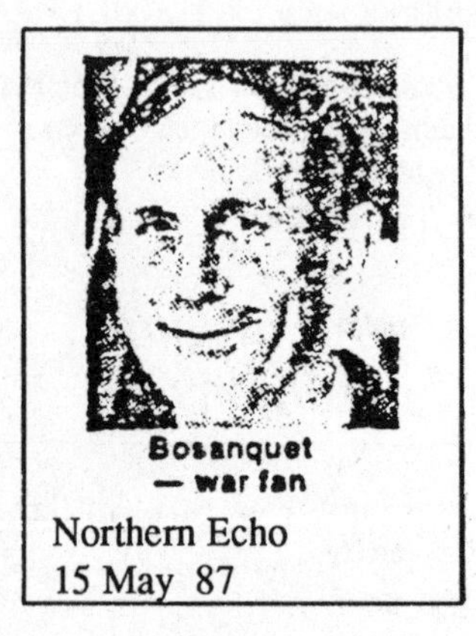

Bosanquet — war fan

Northern Echo 15 May 87

Marks (BMA): Nick Bosanquet is not a doctor, not a manager, not a nurse; he's a chap who knows about figures. (Laughter)

Press Conference 30 Oct 85

We also hear from Professor Tony Culyer of York, Stephen Birch of Sheffield and Martin Buxton of Brunel.

In the last six months York University's centre for health economics has had two peak-time television programmes devoted to its work, and a visit from ubiquitous health minister Mrs Edwina Currie. What has it done to deserve such notoriety?

THES 27 Feb 87

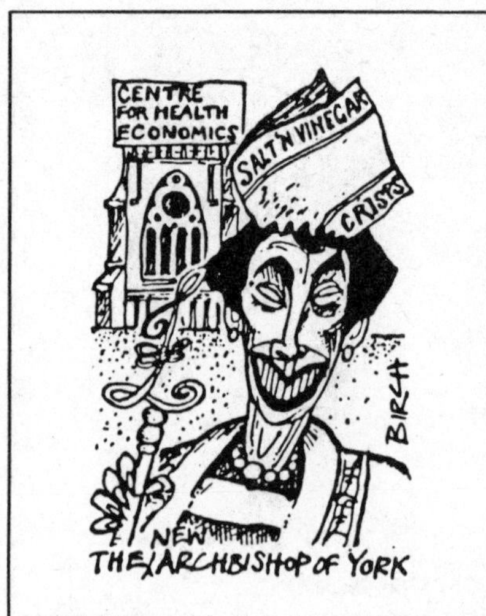

THES 27 Feb 87

A load of QALYs

Guardian 5 Nov 86

Sloppy doctors could face axe

YE Press 16 July 86

Minister fends off York report

YE Press 2 Sept 86

At the heart of the controversy are the harmless-sounding "qalys".

THES 27 Feb 87

WHAT IS a QALY?

Scotsman 5 Jan 87

Watts: As regular listeners to this programme may already know, the word QALY is not a term of abuse nor indeed an expression of endearment but an acronym for quality adjusted life year.

'Medicine Now' BBC Radio 4, 11 Dec 86

. . . the work being carried out by York University in Quality Life Adjusted Years.
Nursing Times and Nursing Mirror 1/7 April 87

The system, based on a scale of "quality of adjusted life years" or QALYs.
Yorkshire Post 3 Sept 86

Cost-benefit analysis would be based on the Qaly (Quality of life years) system.
Guardian 18 June 87

Watts: It's a concept that's arousing interest among health economists but it's controversial. Not everybody loves the QALY.
'Medicine Now' BBC Radio 4, 11 Dec 86

A dubious formula for quantifying your health.
International Management Nov 86

A CONTROVERSIAL METHOD of assessing whether certain patients should receive treatment.
Nursing Times and Nursing Mirror 1/7 April 87

It rhymes with jolly, but it is not. The word looks like a hybrid of a quango and a wally. But it is not that either.
Scotsman 5 Jan 87

This is Quality Assured Life Years, and as a phrase it has all the euphemistic charm of the Final Solution.
New Statesman 30 Jan 87

- it does have an Orwellian ring to it -
Scotsman 5 Jan 87

1987 - a Quality Adjusted Life Year
Therapy Weekly 1 Jan 87

Where do they come from?

The idea is originally American - inevitably -
Scotsman 5 Jan 87

Real people, or administrators anyway, have invented QALYs.
New Statesman 30 Jan 87

Health economists at the University of York have devised [them].
Journal of District Nursing Oct 86

QALYs - quality adjusted life years - were devised by Professor Alan Williams, also at York University, to try to provide some measure of quality of life.
Times 17 June 87

"We need a simple, versatile measure of success which incorporates both life expectancy and quality of life and which reflects the values and ethics of the community served," he wrote as the Quality Adjusted Life Year (QALY) was born.
Scotsman 3 Dec 87

What do they measure?

QALYs measure the outcome of health procedures such as operations, new drugs and so on, in terms of increased life span and improved quality of life.
Therapy Weekly 1 Jan 87

Instead of recording a doctor's clinical assessment of success or failure, they measure how a patient feels and functions after treatment.
Guardian 18 June 87

The QALY approach is a way of measuring the relative value of health benefits; the issue is not how old or sick patients are, but how much better can we make them.

Lancet (Williams) 13 June 87

. . . a system called QUALYS - in which the cost of treatment can be related directly to the patient's resulting quality of life.

Northampton Evening Telegraph 10 June 87

. . . a crude, experimental but nevertheless significant composite measure of the additional life years and improved quality of life of those years generated by certain health procedures.

Journal of District Nursing Oct 86

Health measure

Yorkshire Post 18 Jan 88

It is a handy formula to determine whether it is cost-effective to invest in expensive treatment on someone who is getting old and who won't, in accountant's terms, pay a long-term dividend.

New Statesman 30 Jan 87

"What they really mean, when it comes down to it, is that somebody is saying that your life is not as valuable as somebody else's."

Guardian 18 June 87

Crudely put, they lead to the "one heart transplant = 17 hip replacements" type of equation guaranteed to open medical, financial and ethical cans of worms.

THES 27 Feb 87

The importance of the QALY

Prof. Alan Williams of the University of York argues forcefully for the measurement and valuation of the quality of life, which he hopes will turn out to be "the aspect of health care evaluation which comes historically to be recognised as the great achievement of the last quarter of the twentieth century."

Financial Times 26 June 87

LATE 20th century Man, it seems, engages in the pursuit not of happiness but of QALYs.

Guardian 5 Nov 86

A matter of life or death

Dorset Evening Echo 10 June 87

The debate about the allocation of health resources receives much public discussion these days.

Therapy Weekly 1 Jan 87

At the eye of the storm over NHS funding, doctors are being forced to choose who will live and who will die.

Times 21 Dec 87

Using a person's QALY scores, doctors and economists can determine who will get treatment and who will not. In other words, who will live and who will die.

Scotsman 5 Jan 87

. . . putting life and death on a balance sheet . . .

THES 27 Feb 87

TELEVISION

Observer 12 Oct 86

This Week (ITV, Thursday, 9.30pm) doesn't often extend its subjects into a second week, but with "Who Lives, Who Dies?" they're pulling the stops out, as Jonathan Dimbleby presents what he calls "the agonising dilemma" now facing a National Health Service which is strained to breaking point.

Doctor 16 Oct 86

Dimbleby: A radical new approach to the dilemma of the NHS is afoot. The argument is that on grounds of fairness and finance the NHS must recognise economic reality and face up to an awesome choice.
'This Week', ITV, 16 Oct 86

Painful choices

Nursing Times and Nursing Mirror 1/7 April 87

Hard choices have to be made about who will die and who will live, and in what degree of pain and discomfort.
Geriatric Medicine (Maynard) Nov 87

Many people still find it too shocking to discuss the relative merits of spending money on heart transplants, for example, as opposed to residential care for elderly mentally ill people.
Therapy Weekly 1 Jan 87

Can we afford costly palliatives for the terminally ill? Should we pursue heart transplants while the list for hip operations grows ever longer?
Doctor 16 Oct 86

Should resources be channelled into renal services in the knowledge that without dialysis certain death will follow, the cost being £15,000 per person per year for perhaps ten years? Should resources be channelled into hip replacements whereby people who are housebound not only throw away their crutches but live, laugh and are relieved of the burden of coping with themselves and can once again be concerned for others, at a cost £1,925 per one-off operation?
Nursing Times and Nursing Mirror 1/7 April 87

Hospital dialysis cost £14,000 for every QALY gained - nearly twice as much as the £8,000 per QALY in the case of heart transplants. Hip replacements scored £750 per QALY, a heart bypass operation £2,000 and a heart pacemaker £1,000.
Yorkshire Post 3 Sept 86

Maynard: If we're trying to produce just one year of life with no disability or distress, hips to put it crudely are a much better buy than heart transplants.
'This Week', ITV, 9 Oct 86

Dimbleby: The Centre at York would have the funds diverted from new hearts to new hips.
'This Week', ITV, 9 Oct 86

Fury over prof's kidney call

Northern Echo 3 Sept 86

Prof Alan Williams told the British Association in September that since dialysis was so expensive compared with hip replacement, dialysis should be restrained and the other expanded.

One can only hope that this was careless reporting - and not (literally) careless thinking.
Doctor 9 Oct 86

He said: "We should not shrink from following where the logic of that approach leads us - that hospital dialysis should be restrained and total hip replacement expanded."
Telegraph 3 Sept 86, Guardian 3 Sept 86, Yorkshire Post 3 Sept 86, YE Press (Lead) 2 Sept 86, Bolton Evening News 2 Sept 86, Northern Echo 3 Sept 86, YE Post (Editorial) 4 Sept 86.

"If we want to improve health to benefit as many people as possible we should expand the cheapest treatments until the money runs out."
YE Press 2 Sept 86

NHS: a matter of life and death

Times 17 June 87

The professor admits that hundreds of patients would die if his proposals were adopted and treatment withdrawn.

YE Post 4 Sept 86

But the professor's comments infuriated York mother Jeanette Wells, whose two children suffer from kidney disease.

Northern Echo 3 Sept 86

Mrs Jeanette Wells of Hawthorn Grove said: "If they are talking about cutting back on these services, they are talking about cutting lives."

"For many there is no alternative to dialysis."

Strength

She knows just how valuable dialysis can be, for her courageous nine-year-old daughter Anne has battled against illness throughout her short life.

Anne suffers from a rare metabolic disease which two years ago caused her kidneys to fail.

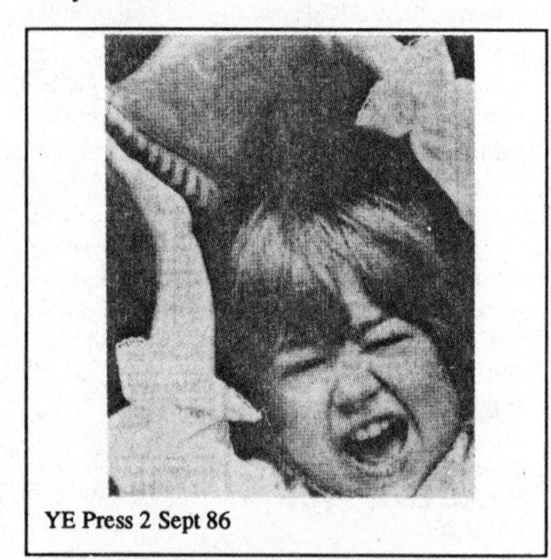

YE Press 2 Sept 86

She was kept alive by dialysis during long months of waiting for a transplant.

The fun-loving youngster had the operation last July and has since gone from strength to strength.

But tragically, her four-year-old brother Andrew also suffers from the rare condition.

Mrs Wells knows his kidneys will also fail and the family will again have to rely on life-saving dialysis treatment.

YE Press 2 Sept 86

Very hard

"When I looked at my daughter playing happily today I just thought what this man said was so very hard," Mrs Wells added.

Northern Echo 3 Sept 86

She added: Angela would probably not be here if it wasn't for dialysis."

"Whie it must be very painful for those people waiting for hip replacements, it is not a matter of life and death."

YE Press 2 Sept 86

The price of life

New Society 2 Jan 87

How do these choices compare with saving the life of a newborn baby whose stay in an intensive care unit costs up to £6,300 per month and can last for as long as 18 months?

Nursing Times and Nursing Mirror 1/7 April 87

BBC's Panorama recently made a programme about "qalys", and then in a second one brought outraged NHS consultants face to face with York centre director Professor Alan Maynard so they could answer him back.

THES 27 Feb 87

[Maynard] proved himself adept at taking the emotion out of health care, as he opted for a little treatment for a lot of patients, rather than concentrating money on saving the life of one premature baby.

Yorkshire Post 11 June 87

Mackintosh (neonatal intensive care): I think the impact [of Maynard's analysis] would be very significant indeed but I think the premise is fallacious to start off with. In neonatal care we don't simply have to consider whether the child dies or survives normally with our treatment. In many instances we provide intensive care for people who would survive without it but would be permanently damaged and therefore a drain on community resources for sixty or seventy years. And that, as far as I can see has not come into the calculations at all . . . .

Dimbleby: Are you putting your ethical, medical heads in the economic sand?

Mackintosh: No. I think we are very cost conscious at the moment. I actually am responsible for the budget in my unit, via the administrator, and I organise that budget as I want within the limits that I'm given but those limits actually restrict me from admitting as many children as I need to admit . . . .

Dimbleby: What would life be like for you in your area if your vision of Professor Maynard's proposals was to become reality?

Mackintosh: I think progress would come to a standstill . . . .

Dimbleby: [So] you have here a senior medical figure [Mackintosh] who is saying that he believes - and he's read your material, understands what you're on about - that you are actually, if you got, as it were, into power, going to halt the advance of medical progress.

Maynard: Yes. I think his fears are ill-founded. I don't think I'm going to get into medical power. What my function is as an economist is to question decision making and try and get better evaluation of decision making.

'This Week', ITV, 16 Oct 86

Dimbleby: The idea that the health service should divert resources away from the intensive care of premature babies outrages the doctors concerned. However the medical profession knows that the question, who lives, who dies, won't go away.

'This Week', ITV, 9 Oct 86

The quack and the dead

Observer 12 Oct 86

THE QUESTION which has been gnawing away all week is briefly put: is it better to be dead or to be a senile dement with double amputation?

Such, according to *Heart of the Matter* (BBC1), are the moral choices daily facing our health administrators under the new QALY system for deciding priorities in NHS treatment.

Observer 12 Oct 86

Maynard: The most emotional health question you can ask is: do you prefer to be dead or to be senile and a double amputee? Now, are there worse cases than death? Many people would rank being senile and a double amputee as worse than death.

'This Week', ITV, 9 Oct 86

A friend of mine died recently. He was a man at the centre of village life. He had had both legs amputated. His last months of life were spent in misery with great pain and without dignity. The amputations gave a few months more existence to a man with a profound faith, anxious to meet his maker.

Nursing Times and Nursing Mirror 1/7 April 87

I suppose the simple answer the quacks want is dead. But not necessarily. Say your senile dementia was so advanced you didn't realise that you were also a double amputee? Say you thought you had the odd hand or a foot? Say you did have the odd hand or foot? How many extra points for those?

Observer 12 Oct 86

No rationale in medical rationing

Doctor 9 Oct 86

Professor Alan Maynard from the University said life or death choices were already being made in various parts of health care.

Belfast Newsletter 13 Oct 86

Researchers at the Centre for Health Economics at York University have devoted much time to reminding ministers, the public and health workers that such decisions are made (often in a very arbitrary way) that it is difficult to foresee a future where such decisions will not be necessary and that it is vital to devise ways of making them in a more rational manner.

Therapy Weekly 1 Jan 87

Ideally care would be rationed in the NHS according to the patients' ability to benefit, in terms of increased duration and quality of life. In reality, of course, the rationing is based on implicit and crude criteria rather than explicit measurement of outcomes.

HSJ (Maynard) 3 Nov 87

People were getting budgets because they shouted loudly and waved shrouds and were generally emotional.

Belfast Newsletter 13 Oct 86

[Williams] said: "The present system is too heavily influenced by dramatic cases, and too little by thinking calmly and rationally about our priorities and objectives."

Yorkshire Post 3 Sept 86

Mr Martin Buxton said: "It is not acceptable any longer to ignore information on costs or benefits where such information exists and to revert to emotional appeal, rhetoric or political expediency."

Times 3 Sept 86

But the general secretary of the National Union of Public Employees, Mr Rodney Bickerstaffe told the London conference: "There are resources going on many decisions outside the Health Service while our people are dying.

"There are thousands of children like little Ben Hardwick who die unnecessarily.

"We need a caring Government to make a caring society . . . .

"This may be rhetoric but you can't sit here and talk about who will die. I believe we need rhetoric and emotion."

YE Press 3 June 86

These things are rarely as simple as professors would like to pretend.

Observer 12 Oct 86

Health care rationing: let's be explicit and systematic

Geriatric Medicine Nov 87

What QALYs are attempting to do is to bring a rationality into decision making about priorities.

HSJ 30 Nov 86

What cost-quality judgements do is bring it out in the open.

THES 27 Feb 87

[They offer] an open and explicit and rational frame-work.

Belfast Newsletter 13 Oct 86

Choices made by the health service would be more humane and efficient 'and not based merely on political pressure or the quest for technological advancement'.

Nursing Times and Nursing Mirror 16 Nov 86

"What we are saying we would like is explicit rationing criteria - and a

public debate about it," said Professor Maynard.

Belfast Newsletter 13 Oct 86

Sadly, this initiative has already met with hostility, and not only from the medical profession but from the public who find it hard to accept that no health service can have unlimited funds.

Nursing Times and Nursing Mirror 1/7 April 87

"The man in the street gets very concerned when we turn around and say because you have reached 'X' age you cannot have 'Y' treatment because it is not cost-effective."

YE Press 2 Sept 86

There cannot have been a more chilling example of the coldness of calculators . . .

YE Post 4 Sept 86

Chilling

YE Post 4 Sept 86

Dimbleby: In Britain the proposal that economics should be applied to matters of life and death provokes bitter hostility.

'This Week', ITV, 16 Oct 86

WHAT is a life worth? That may seem a question for philosophers but increasingly, and to some people unacceptably, it is becoming the preserve of health economists.

Scotsman 3 Dec 86

[QALYs] are "positively dangerous and morally indefensible," [said] Dr John Harris, research director of Manchester University's Centre for Social Ethics and Policy.

Scotsman 3 Dec 86

QALYs, I fear, are the same old guesses and prejudices dressed in impressive new clothes which make them dangerously attractive to those who have the unenviable job of managing the NHS.

Guardian 5 Nov 86

CONTROVERSIAL

Nursing Times and Nursing Mirror 18 Nov 86

The controversial quality adjusted life year (QALY) has so far won few places in the hearts of those who allocate NHS resources.

HSJ 27 Nov 87

The study . . . received a sceptical response from Mr Stuart Ingham, York Health Authority's district general manager.

Basis

He said: "It is an increasingly useful tool in discussions on where we put our money, but at the end of the day it cannot be the only basis on which you make your decision. You have to look at all the subjective and semi-political considerations as well."

YE Press 2 Sept 86

Prof. Williams also came under fire from John White, unit administrator at York District Hospital.

"We do our best here to respond to the clinical needs of all our patients," he said.

Northern Echo 3 Sept 86

His proposal was condemmed by the British Medical Association. "There's a lot of pseudo-scientific jargon about Qalys," said Dr John Lynch, a member of its general practitioners' committee.

Guardian 18 June 87

Doctor: We know, though, and you must know that measuring quality of life is not just a simple index; it's extremely difficult to measure, and to measure it reproducibly.

'This Week', ITV, 16 Oct 86

QALYs are of little or no benefit when applied to individual patients. Indeed, they were never intended to be. Since

doctors undertake the rationing process at the level of patients, they see QALYs as irrelevant to their work. It is no use offering a patient with end-stage renal failure a hip replacement if his hips are perfectly normal. It is no use asking a cardiac surgeon to undertake hip replacements since he will not have the necessary expertise.
Lancet 14 March 87

Asked if he had support from the medical profession, Professor Maynard said:
"There is increasing medical support beginning to come from the medical profession because they do need to get his criteria for they know they are rationing resources, deciding who should live and who should die.
Belfast Newsletter 13 Oct 86

Towards a more refined QALY

HSJ 27 Nov 86

Professor Maynard admitted yesterday that existing Qaly measurements were poor, but they should be improved, not thrown out, he argued.
Guardian 18 June 87

Our challenge is "If you say our measures are crude, we agree. But don't just dismiss them, because if we dismiss them we are back to shroud-waving."
THES 27 Feb 87

North Western RHA using QALYs to improve quality

Public Finance and Accountancy Nov 86

Principal Assistant Regional Treasurer Tim Scott said that North Western's joint project with the CHE has confirmed the potential of QALYs as an adjunct to decision-making, and he hoped the new report would help to focus the QALY debate and dispel some of the misinformation which he felt surrounded the measure.
Public Finance and Accountancy Nov 86

Professor Maynard: "It is going to cause a debate hopefully coherent. Obviously doctors may want to make it incoherent to defend their own economic interests. I hope that will not happen. I hope it will be rational and cool, and that the general public can contribute to it."
Belfast Newsletter 13 Oct 86

He conceded that doctors might not welcome the plan: "We tried it in the North-western health region in 1985 and 1986, but we did not get very far. We ran into opposition from the medical profession. They did not like the quality-of-life measurements."
Guardian 18 June 87

It is this inherent human foible - that nobody wants to take the hardest decisions - that has prevented QALYs from getting a wider hearing.
Times 17 June 87

WHO DECIDES?

The proposal is that these "scores" will be arrived at by "doctors and economists working together." What is not clear is who decides what "quality" means. Nor what constitutes "perfect wellbeing." Nor who decides what, in this context, "utility" means. Certainly it is not suggested anywhere in the document that the patient, or the patient's relatives, should make any contribution to this process.
Scotsman 5 June 87

The big unanswered question is, who is going to make the choices? Any doctor will tell you that an informal system of rationing exists today. The health economists want to make it formal, structured, clear to all. Most people who feel that they could afford to do so would want to control the process themselves. Must the poor forever have such choices made for them? We will only begin to get serious

answers to such questions when the Government turns aside from the political auction on NHS spending and brings forward the fundamental dilemmas for public debate.
Financial Times 26 June 87

I was with Mr Sells and Dr John Harris, a senior lecturer in philosophy at Manchester University, who thought that a lottery would be better than pretending we had a way to decide who was valuable.
The Tablet 11 Oct 86

Money or life

Belfast Newsletter 13 Oct 86

In economic terms the professor may be talking sound business sense. But, thank God, the saving of life in the final analysis is not in the hands of the people with the calculators.

If that were so, the "quality of life" for us all would be under permanent strain.
YE Post 4 Sept 86

If the only decisions were economic ones, then it would tend to be accountants, not doctors, who made them.
The Tablet 11 Oct 86

Maynard: Are we making the right sort of decisions? We're not going to make the decisions for you. What we're trying to do is to give you evaluative information about outcomes and about costs so as to improve and assist your decision making. Thankfully, I don't have to make those decisions.
'This Week', ITV, 16 Oct 86

At present, he claimed, doctors and politicians were making many of these fundamental decisions.
Belfast Newsletter 13 Oct 86

Mackintosh: But if in fact government and health care economists are going to dictate [the size of my budget] then society has to come in to making this decision. Not politicians, not economists, but society itself.
'This Week', ITV, 16 Oct 86

Clearly, it depends on who you ask, and most people would find it an intolerable choice to take. Who will decide these things?
Scotsman 5 Jan 87

a game of chance

Times 21 Dec 87

The author and broadcaster, Dr Michael O'Donnell sees it differently. "People who make vital decisions on their assessment of the quality of other people's lives are playing a real life version of the game in which you decide whom to throw from the gondola of an overloaded balloon. In real life poets, artists, "wets", the old and the infirm will be the first to go and if the game lasts long enough it will probably end with a gondola full of generals."
Scotsman 3 Dec 86

It could be a question from one of those new-style board games so popular this Christmas: "If you had one place left in your lifeboat and could decide to save the life either of a 17-year-old girl or a 34-year-old mother of two children, who would you choose?"
Times 21 Dec 87

Health care roulette

Guardian 5 Nov 86

Say that three patients of the same age presented simultaneously with end-stage renal failure: one a professor of health service economics (or a general manager or a consultant), who had plenty of outside activities; the second unemployed, whose social activities alternated between the television and the pub; the third mentally subnormal. All three would have different qualities of life, not measurable on the scale devised by Rosser and Williams,[4,6] but for all three the same number of QALYs would be generated by treatment at a given cost. Who therefore should be chosen for the single dialysis place? Should it be left to the arguing powers of the patient and his family, the prejudices of the doctor, some measurements of value to society, or to the Government's objective of improving care for the mentally subnormal? Experience in the real world tells us that the first person in this particular queue would receive treatment. But is this just? Or should selection for this treatment be based on a lottery that gives everyone an equal chance and avoids any form of prejudice?[11]

Lancet 14 March 87

O'Donnell is advocating the use of lotteries to decide who shall get the benefits of health care.

This is a breathtakingly radical solution to the problems that have been exercising medical scientists and clinicians over centuries.

Professor Alam Williams.
Institute of Social and Economic Research,
University of York.

Guardian 12 Nov 86

Williams: If there was a choice for say heroic surgery between a 95 year old terminal cancer case . . . or a young motorcyclist . . . who has another 60 years of active life ahead . . . is he saying they should enter the lottery on the same terms?

'Medicine Now', BBC Radio 4, 11 Dec 86

Life or death decision

Northamptonshire Evening Telegraph 10 June 87

TV doctor Miriam Stoppard turns game show host tonight . . . with prizes of either life or death.

Miriam invites her studio audience to decide the fate of two hospital patients in The Life and Death Game.

Northamptonshire Evening Telegraph 10 June 87

At the forefront of this is Professor Alan Maynard, a health economist from York University, who agreed to play God for the benefit of last night's programme so that his views could gain more publicity.

Yorkshire Post 11 June 87

"Some people may think it trivialises an important issue. But if it brings it to the attention of more people then it's worthwhile."

Northamptonshire Evening Telegraph 10 June 87

One member of the audience described Professor Maynard's views as a load of codswallop, but a near majority were impressed by his arguments.

Yorkshire Post 11 June 87

Diagnosing where the doctor is wrong

Daily Express 17 July 86

So far it has been the consultants who have berated Maynard and the York centre. But work now under way on the general practitioner service will be equally controversial.

THES 27 Feb 87

radical solutions

General Practitioner 17 Oct 86

Professor Alan Maynard is building a reputation for advocating radical solutions to the future of primary health care in Britain.

General Practitioner 17 Oct 86

Prof. Maynard said general practice was in need of "radical reform."

Doctor 24 July 86

Professor Alan Maynard's radical proposals include year-long contracts between patients and their family doctor, and National Health Service payments out of which the general practitioner would provide comprehensive health care for the patient, including hospitalization.

Times 14 July 86

He said: 'You may think we are arguing about the obvious but our activities are regarded as extremely radical and extremely provocative by some powerful self-interest groups in the health care market.
'It is these groups that need to be persuaded - along with politicians - to improve the health care system.'

Hospital Doctor 11 Sept 86

Ethical need to monitor doctors

HSJ 16 Oct 86

At present, according to Maynard, the country spends £2.5 billion on GPs and the drugs they prescribe, and no one knows what they do.

THES 27 Feb 87

Professor Maynard criticised GPs' free role to run their practices. 'Nobody knows what GPs do', he said, 'but what research has been done throws an interesting light on the matter.'

General Practitioner 6 Dec 86

He pointed to a recent survey which claimed that GPs spend only an average 15 hours a week with patients, and called for a shake-up of doctors' duties.

YE Press 3 June 86

Profession puts on uncaring face

Doctor 24 July 86

Family doctors' attitudes to their patients were also attacked by Prof. Alan Maynard, director of York University's centre for health economics.

He told the meeting "Sometimes primary care seems to be organised more for the convenience, or perhaps the leisure, of GPs than the interest of patients."

Doctor 24 July 86

Sack urged for the duffer GPs

YE Press 5 Nov 86

Prof. Maynard, of York University, told the meeting that the inflexibility of doctors' contracts was one of the major obstacles to better management of resources in the health service . . . .

Doctors' contracts would, eventually, have to become more flexible if the NHS was to survive in the market place.

Hospital Doctor 11 Sept 86

"Short-term contracts rather than jobs for life may be consistent with efficiency, if inconsistent with professional restrictive practices."

Daily Telegraph 13 Oct 86

Medical groups 'halt advance of health care'

Hospital Doctor 11 Sept 86

Doctors, he said, had sectional interests and could not, on the whole, be persuaded to take an overall view.

"If you sit on a health authority like I do you will know that trying to control these people or find out

what they are doing is virtually impossible."
Hospital Doctor 11 Sept 86

The nonsense of doctors' contracts

HSJ 19/26 Dec 85

A YORK University professor's proposal family doctors should have their contracts reviewed every four years got a cool reception from the British Medical Association yesterday....

The spokesman said: "Prof. Maynard holds no responsibility for patients whatsoever and we think it is surprising that he was holding forth in that arena."

Professor Maynard . . . said resistance to his proposals was to be expected.

Northern Echo 16 July 86

Letters

Doctors should have long term contracts . . .

HSJ 23 Jan 86

. . . but what about professors?

HSJ 23 Jan 86

Alan Maynard comments: We have to meet our customers' needs or we will cease to exist. If we fail to satisfy our customers' needs I look forward to joining medical colleagues, who have failed similarly, in the dole queue.

HSJ 23 Jan 86

Doctors' salaries 'waste of cash'

Yorkshire Post 13 Oct 86

Health service doctors are overpaid, and many of their routine duties could be performed just as well by nurses, according to a York University report . . . .

As a result, more and more of the NHS budget is going into the pockets of Britain's doctors.

YE Press 15 Oct 86

Use nurses, says report

Yorkshire Post 13 Oct 86

"Do you actually need skilled nurses in all the roles you have now?

"One of the biggest manpower demands now is in geriatric wards where old people need bathing and taking to the loo. You don't need skilled nurses for that. Maybe you could get by with one nurse at the head of a less-qualified team."

Yorkshire Post 18 Jan 88

A spokeswoman for the British Medical Association last night dismissed the possibility of widespread substitution of nurses for doctors. "No patient in Britain is complaining that there are too many doctors around" she said.

Daily Telegraph 13 Oct 86

Efficiency

She pointed to a report by the National Association of Health Authorities which says that hospitals are overstretched because of an acute shortage of doctors.

YE Press 13 Oct 86

Playing the doctors' numbers game

General Practitioner 17 Oct 86

Now the head of York University's centre for health economics has come forward with a series of controversial proposals on future planning of doctors' numbers.

General Practitioner 17 Oct 86

Co-author Mr Stephen Birch explained: "We are not saying we have too many doctors at the moment."
YE Press 13 Oct 86

More family doctors for Yorks call
YE Press 23 Oct 86

Family doctor services distributed 'unfairly'
Independent 23 Oct 86

Economist Prof. Alan Maynard told the meeting that improvements would require drastic changes in the status of doctors and were fiercely resisted by organisations including the BMA.
Hospital Doctor 11 Sept 86

Criticised
YE Press 13 Oct 86

The report's conclusions have been criticised by the British Medical Association.

A spokesman said: "We have the lowest number of doctors per head of population than any other country throughout Europe except Greece.

"To say that we have too many, and that they are overpaid, is beyond comprehension."
YE Press 13 Oct 86

"It is an enthusiastic suggestion and society needs its enthusiasts because occasionally they come up with a good idea. But this is not one of them," said Dr Peter Kielty, a British Medical Association negotiator for family doctors.

"We have 28,000 family doctors and on this plan 7,000 a year would have to be assessed. It would mean appointing 100 doctors as full-time assessors, and their salaries plus bureaucratic overheads would cost millions," he said. "The only clear thing is that it would cost a fortune."
Daily Express 17 July 86

The academics say that the lack of systematic planning and forecasting 'may reflect the power and convenience to the medical profession rather than the interests of NHS patients or taxpayers.'
General Practitioner 17 Oct 86

But this view, and indeed the main thrust of Professor Maynard's formula for change, is regarded by General Medical Services Committee member Dr Jim Milligan as an effort to catch the government's eye.

Dr Milligan makes the point that GPs are equally capable of providing a set of radical alternatives to the indecision-making that has bedevilled the NHS manpower structure.
General Practitioner 17 Oct 86

Prof. Maynard said: "I bear the wounds of an attack from the BMA - clearly they were not prepared to consider that."
Hospital Doctor 11 Sept 86

Although his views may not be palatable to GPs, they receive much attention from the DHSS and ministers alike.
General Practitioner 17 Oct 86

Health as a political football
Sunday Times 12 Oct 86

It is this central funding relationship between Government and the health service which is awry and must be corrected. A good starting point would be for both sides to start talking the same language in terms of health economics.
HSJ 31 Oct 85

Mackintosh: The wrong premise in the first place is that there aren't enough resources. And there aren't enough

resources as they are given at the moment. But the gross national product put into health care in this country is despicably low compared to the rest of Europe and the States.
'This Week', ITV, 16 Oct 86

How does the NHS perform in relation to the benefit objective that Mrs Thatcher espoused at the 1982 Conservative Party Conference, and which has been reiterated regularly since then?
HSJ 2 June 86

NHS cash

HSJ 24 July 86

Nick Bosanquet, of the Centre for Health Economics at the University of York, in an unprecedented link up with the Institute of Health Services Management (IHSM), the British Medical Association (BMA) and the Royal College of Nursing (RCN), has published a paper on the outlook for public expenditure on the NHS.
HSJ 31 Oct 85

They are seeking a doubling of the Government's planned real growth in expenditure from 1-2 per cent a year for the next three years.
HSJ 31 Oct 85

Missing cash—case proven

HSJ 24 July 86

Marks: What this report as far as I am concerned has done is to produce factual evidence of what anecdotally I know to be true: that there's not enough money spent on the health service.
Press Conference 30 Oct 85

It's the figures that count

HSJ 31 Oct 85

The IHSM, the BMA, and the RCN hope that the work of the Centre for Health Economics will be seen as an objective, non-partisan study on which agreement can be reached between the funders, providers and consumers of health care on planning and managing the NHS into the 1990s.
RCN, BMA, IHSM Press Release 28 Oct 85

Journalist: There have been a lot of figures flying around the last few months about what the spending is and what resources actually are. Do you hope that this report will sort of be seen as an objective comment on the situation and will be sort of the last word, in terms of the argument, or do you think the Government will now say No, this isn't the situation, you've got it wrong?
Jarrold (IHSM): Very good point. Of course our answer would be Yes, we do hope to be regarded as objectively the last word but I think there's no chance whatsoever of that because I think, as both John [Marks] and Trevor [Clay]have said, the NHS is now firmly at the centre of the political stage and there is no doubt that the statements of the kind that we have made today will be answered and challenged vigorously by those whose interest it is to discredit them . . . so I think today is not the end of the figures being thrown about . . . .
Marks: I'm sure it won't be the last word, it can't be. We will produce figures which we happen to believe are objective. The government will produce figures which it thinks are genuine and there will be a difference. (Laughter) We think that ours are impartial.
Press Conference 30 Oct 85

Lies, damned lies, and NHS statistics

HSJ 23 Jan 86

Unpalatably, what Nick Bosanquet reveals is that most of the statements on NHS finance emerging from the Department of Health's press office are little more than pie in the sky.

HSJ 31 Oct 85

In the 2 per cent debate the Minister's main opponent was Nick Bosanquet of the Centre for Health Economics, University of York.

HSJ 29 May 86

Ministers admit need for 2 per cent NHS growth

HSJ 23 Jan 86

Nick Bosanquet said that it was certainly a 'significant statement'.

HSJ 23 Jan 86

Minister corrects 'errors' in spending estimates

HSJ 30 Jan 86

The Minister has said that although he accepts a number of points in Mr Bosanquet's report he wants to correct some major errors in the original document.

Mr Hayhoe said that he agreed, as the report suggests, that health authority services need to grow by about 2 per cent a year in order to meet the pressures they face.

'But I must emphasise that it is services and not expenditure that need to grow by 2 per cent.'

The Minister said the report ignored the contribution made by greater efficiency.

HSJ 30 Jan 86

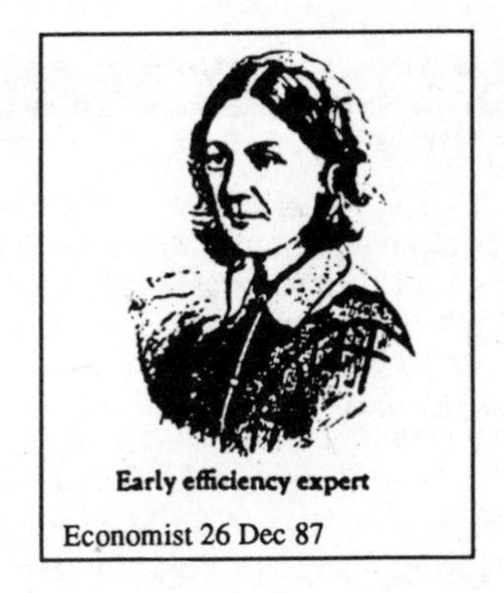

Early efficiency expert

Economist 26 Dec 87

While it is difficult to be original with an exhortation to greater efficiency, a detailed examination of the funding aspects of health care, while the Government's star chamber is making crucial financial decisions, is extremely apposite.

HSJ 31 Oct 85

Mrs Thatcher urged to pump £300m into NHS

Pulse 6 Sept 86

The appeal was contained in a strongly-worded message sent to Prime Minister Mrs Thatcher pointing out that despite Government pledges there had been no significant increase in NHS funding for the previous four years.

The concern of health professionals was revealed at a press conference at

the BMA on Monday which heard of evidence supplied by the Centre for Health Economics based at York University.

Pulse 6 Sept 86

'Stop the NHS cuts'

Pulse 6 Sept 86

The report was commissioned from York University's Centre for Health Economics by the Institute of Health Service Managers, the British Medical Association and the Royal College of Nursing.

Public Finance and Accountancy 5 Sept 86

Prepared by Prof Alan Maynard and Dr Nick Bosanquet, of York University's Centre for Health Economics, it endorses the findings of the first report published in October 1985.

The authors conclude that at least a two per cent increase in NHS funding is essential.

Doctor 11 Sept 86

DOCTORS, nurses and health managers claim to have provided Health Secretary Norman Fowler with the ammunition he needs to talk more money out of the Treasury.

Doctor 11 Sept 86

But the Government hit back in a statement from Health Minister, Mr. Norman Fowler.

He says spending in real terms under the Tories has increased by 24 per cent since 1978/79.

Savings

Mr Fowler said "In other words, the two per cent increase has already been achieved."

YE Press 2 Sept 86

Mr Bosanquet added: "The two per cent needed has not been achieved, even allowing for cost improvements in the key hospital and community health services.

"I must admit the Government response has been disappointing."

YE Press 2 Sept 86

But since recent rumours that political pressures were causing the Government to rethink its stance on NHS spending the debate took on another dimension.

HSJ 29 May 86

pay-out

Doctor 11 Sept 86

HEALTH SERVICE WELCOMES WINDFALL FROM MINISTERS

Nursing Times and Nursing Mirror 1 Nov 86

Mr Nick Bosanquet, senior research fellow at the York University centre for health economics and author of a recent report on NHS expenditure, said last night that Mr Fowler may have done enough to avert a serious crisis.

Guardian 2 June 86

Prof Alan Maynard: "Significant cash problems."

YE Press 3 June 86

Professor Maynard admitted there did seem to have been a real increase in National Health Service resources.

'But it is inadequate to meet the demands the government articulates each year in the public expenditure white paper.'

More money alone was not the answer. 'We have to divert resources to enable the service to perform more efficiently.'

HSJ 2 June 86

FROM AN IVORY TOWER

HSJ (Maynard column heading) 1987

Dimbleby: Professor Maynard is not an isolated voice. His team at York is financed by government and its work is given close attention by the DHSS.
'This Week', ITV, 16 Oct 86

Prof. Maynard told Social Services Secretary, Mr Norman Fowler, and Health Minister, Mr Barney Hayhoe, that university academic staff no longer have the security of jobs for life, so why should GPs?
YE Press 16 July 86

Ministers are known to favour the plan, originally drawn up by the York University health economist, Professor Alan Maynard. But it was considered too radical to be included in the green paper on GP services.
Guardian 19 June 86

But Maynard argues that the government frequently gets advice from York that it does *not* want to hear, and that the civil servants at least in the DHSS who commission research are open-minded about the answers.
THES 27 Feb 87

Health ministers have been careful to keep out of the debate. The DHSS has been equally wary.
Times 17 June 87

The professor's work is funded by government by the Department of Health. He guessed that his views were going to prevail in the debate.
Belfast Newsletter 13 Oct 86

Maynard's point is that the information is neutral: economics is simply a tool to understand what is happening. Policy decisions on using that information are still in the hands of doctors and policy-makers.
THES 27 Feb 87

"What we essentially regard ourselves doing is informing policy-makers."
THES 27 Feb 87

Policy makers 'prefer ignorance and prejudice'

Hospital Doctor 12 June 86

"They do not wish to be confused by facts about the real world, preferring to remain in a dream world of ignorance and prejudice," he told the conference.
Hospital Doctor 12 June 86

Efficiency options are fudged by policymakers and politicians alike because they would involve such things as explicit prioritisation and confronting the monopoly power of provider groups, especially clinicians.
HSJ (Maynard) 3 Nov 87

This cowardice by policymakers is a major threat to the survival of the NHS.
HSJ (Maynard) 3 Nov 87

Sometimes we bring good news and sometimes we bring bad.
THES 27 Feb 87

Prof Maynard . . . failure.
Hospital Doctor 12 June 86

The pursuit of policies to equalise health-care expenditure is pathetic . . . .

Such action would be politically difficult because sectional interests would lose out . . . . Neither the present government nor the Labour opposition

seems capable of confronting these problems as there are perhaps too many marginal constituencies at stake.
HSJ (Maynard) 3 Nov 87

'The government does lots of nice crude calculations, saying we need a 1 per cent increase in expenditure to meet the demands from more elderly.

'That's a very dangerous argument by the DHSS, because its statistical basis is less than robust.'
HSJ 2 June 86

"The Government spends a lot of money on collecting information for its Hospital Activity Analysis. But it's a joke. It only gives information on expenditure and on doing things. But no-one in the NHS knows the cost of anything and the data on outcomes is lousy."
Yorkshire Post 18 Jan 88

As for current data such as the generation of performance indicators, Professor Maynard dismissed them as useless.
Laboratory News 26 June 87

Health studies 'quick and dirty'
Laboratory News 26 June 87

Studies such as those to be carried on NHS pathology are described by Professor Maynard as "quick and dirty" appraisals for agencies requiring "instant wisdom."
Laboratory News 26 June 87

"But there's an increasing awareness of the power of very simple economic techniques in illuminating what's going on in the health service."
THES 27 Feb 87

are health economists a sufficient answer?
Nature 18 June 87

Professor Maynard believes that government should turn to the research community to provide answers to policy problems.
Laboratory News 26 June 87

The DHSS trains just six health economists a year to deal with a health care system that consumes £20 billion a year.
Laboratory News 26 June 87

"The government's attitude to health economics is a very simple one—that of cost containment. Economists take a much longer term view."
Laboratory News 26 June 87

'Be quick and dirty' researchers told
HSJ 31 Oct 85

Researchers are warned of perfectionism and urged towards 'quick and dirty' studies in a new discussion paper from Tony Culyer, professor at the Centre for Health Economics, York.
HSJ 31 Oct 85

The Centre for Health Economics has been commissioned by the IHSM to provide a detailed answer to the white paper (see page 96) which will probably be available in about a fortnight.
HSJ 23 Jan 86

Professor Culyer also urges health economists to adopt a higher profile . . .
HSJ 31 Oct 85

But how could you seriously hope to measure—with the . . . conditions and social circumstances . . . possibly varying enormously—without invidious comparisons being made?
Yorkshire Post 18 Jan 88

"Yes, there is a chance you would get trial-by-media. So, we can either do what we do now and stay in ignorance, or work out a civilised means of assessing performance."
Yorkshire Post 18 Jan 88

And, to round it all off, Bobby rose again from the dead (*Dallas*, BBC1). Happily, this appears not yet to be available on the NHS. Goodness knows how many QALYs a resurrection scores.
Observer 12 Oct 86

Meanwhile at the other end of the University of York campus, away from the bright lights of the media . . .

THE OTHER YORK: HEALTH ECONOMICS UNDER THE MICROSCOPE

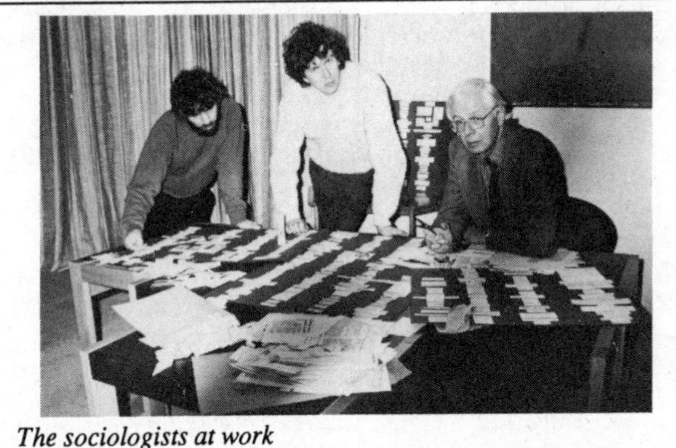
The sociologists at work

Ever wondered about the blue-suited pundits with the calculators, who want life and death decisions made on economic grounds? A new study of health economists reveals all.

Our reporters investigate

SOCIOLOGY STAR RISING

If York has a reputation in health economics it is also fast becoming known for its sociology of science. York Vice-Chancellor, Berrick Saul, in launching a recent appeal for more social science funding at York said: "The University Grants Committee has recognised York's achievement in the social sciences by awarding its elusive 'star rating' for out-standing work to two key departments, Economics and Social Policy, and also to the Sociology Department for its work on sociology of science". As yet largely unknown outside the academic community, York's sociologists of science are set to make a wider impact with their latest study of health economics.

PRIZE WINNING PROF

What is sociology of science? According to York's prize-winning professor, Michael Mulkay, it is "The discipline which examines how science works and thus enables scientists to know themselves." Mulkay and his team are known for their work on physics and biology, but for the last three years they have been turning their spotlight onto the social science of health economics. In view of all the media attention that Professor Maynard and co. have attracted it would seem a natural target for the sociologists. But Professor Mulkay denies that the media attention had anything to do with the choice. "The health economists have only really been in the public eye over the last couple of years. When we started our research we had no idea that health economics would get this kind of attention." York's controversial Centre for Health Economics figures prominently in the sociologists' study but they are anxious to point out that health economics is much more than just what goes on at York. They also say they have looked at the use made of health economics by medics and NHS bureaucrats. While the health economists have been gaining public attention, Mulkay and his team have preferred to keep a low profile. However, this may all change with the publication of the team's controversial new book.

RADICAL CLAIMS

Mulkay and his colleagues Dr Trevor Pinch and Dr Malcolm Ashmore advance several radical new ideas about health economics in the book. The most controversial of all is that health economists are really just another sectional group within the health-care system, who in essence are every bit as self-interested as doctors and administrators. The only difference is that the health economists claim a special privilege of neutrality and objectivity for their recommendations. But, say the sociologists, this God-like status is unwarranted. "While health economists berate others for indulging in shroud waving, emotion and rhetoric, they themselves hide behind the shroud of objectivity."

DILEMMA

Health economists differ from other scientists studied by the York sociologists because they set out to change the world. "They want to put their ideas into practice by influencing decision making in the NHS." Most academic researchers can maintain a front of objectivity and disinterest because they work in ivory towers. In contrast, the health economists get involved in the messy world of human affairs in the attempt to get their principles adopted as the new basis for NHS rationing.

To have any effect the health economists must get the ear of the government and the public at large, as well as NHS personnel. They use the media at every opportunity to get their message across. To attract media attention, they issue press releases, send memoranda to Government, and invite the press to their conferences. Best known of them all is York's Professor Alan Maynard, who regularly appears as a pundit on BBC Radio 4's popular "Today" programme. Maynard has also appeared on three peak-time TV documentaries about his work.

But jumping on the media band-wagon can involve dangers, warn the sociologists. The dilemma for the health economists is that every appearance in the media makes them appear less disinterested and more like all the other NHS pressure groups constantly seeking the public lime light. "This is the hidden cost or disbenefit of using the media" Dr Ashmore told us.

SIMPLE CHOICES

The sociologists have discovered that health economists' arguments in the media tend to follow a standard pattern. Remember Alan Maynard's famous 1986 confrontation with Jonathan Dimbleby on ITV's "This Week"? Maynard started off by claiming that decision-making in the NHS is irrational, based as it is on ignorance, political self-interest and emotional appeal - "shroud waving" as Maynard likes to refer to it. He then contrasted this irrational world with the system of explicit rationing based on the objective appraisal of costs and benefits advocated by health economists. "This offers an open, explicit and rational framework" said Maynard, as he went on to dramatize the situation by pointing to the hard choices that have to be made: for instance, between being dead and being a double-amputee with senile dementia - according to Maynard this is the "most emotional health question you can ask". But how realistic is this choice?

Not very realistic perhaps, but according to

the sociologists that doesn't matter as much as the way in which the claims are presented. "Research on political rhetoric has shown that the most effective speakers always present their messages either in lists of three or as a contrast. Maynard, like Thatcher and Scargill, is good at both." Another hard choice favoured by health economists in their media presentations is that between hip replacements and kidney dialysis. This is a particular favourite with Maynard's colleague Professor Alan Williams. Having dramatized and simplified complicated issues of resource allocation into this single choice, it is then shown on grounds of economic fairness why that choice should be made differently. The upshot is to recommend more hip operations and less dialysis.

BOGUS NEUTRALITY?

The health economists always present their own information and criteria for choice as being neutral. When pushed they sometimes deny that they are making specific recommendations and claim that they merely wish to inform policy makers and start a public debate. As Maynard told Dimbleby "I hope the debate will be explicit, rational and cool". If challenged that they are playing God they say that choices are already being made but on implicit and irrational grounds. If their proposals run into resistance it is because those who oppose them are corrupted by self-interest. Maynard's favourite target group is doctors - he is known in certain circles as the Doctor-Bashing Professor.

HAVING IT BOTH WAYS

Professor Mulkay and his colleagues point out that the health economists' ruse of posing as neutral experts is increasingly being rumbled. People who are familiar with medical decision-making are sceptical that an explicit principle of rationing can be found which represents everyone's best interests. Consequently, health economists' interventions are increasingly open to challenge on the grounds that they, too, are interest-based. Economists are seen as Thatcherite cost-cutters or mere attention seekers. Ironically, their stated desire to promote an open rational debate has also back-fired in that their proposals have been greeted in some quarters by a tirade of anger, abuse and emotion. The outrage following Maynard's first confrontation with Dimbleby led ITV to produce a second programme in which senior medical consultants had an opportunity to respond. Promotion of the ubiquitous QALY (Quality Assumed Life Year) has produced the strongest reaction in the media - the health economists have been characterized as unfeeling calculators proposing Nazi-like solutions to matters of life and death. The paradox which the York sociologists point out is that the health economists try to argue for objectivity and rationality in one of the most emotional and irrational forums available - namely the prime-time TV programme. "The health economists face some hard choices. Either they ignore the media and their message has no effect or they use the media and then pay the penalty" is how Dr Pinch described matters.

In an atmosphere where statistics are routinely bandied around and contested by all sorts of interest groups, it seems unlikely that the health economists' figures will prevail merely on the grounds of their supposed disinterestedness and neutrality. To believe as much would be naive in the extreme. However, this is the sort of naivety which the health economists seem at times to display. The debate over Bosanquet's and Maynard's recent reports recommending a 2% increase in funding for the NHS illustrates this point. Their figures - unsurprisingly - received short shrift from Government health ministers and yet Bosanquet was reported to be "disappointed" at the Government's response.

MEDIA RISKS

The York sociologists' point is that playing the media game entails risk. Misquotation and misinformation are rampant. A notorious example is the acronym "QALY". At least six different versions of what it means are circulating in the press. Other dangers are the media's use of eye-catching headlines; their preference for dramatic heart-pulling portrayals of dying children; and their use of guilt-by-association - the QALY, for example, has been described as "Orwellian." The danger in trying to use the media, is that the media will use you. And, of course, the health economists' work is reported in different ways in papers with different political slants and readerships.

PIN-UP PROFESSOR

One very clear result of lengthy exposure in the media is trivialization - the 'pin-up professor' phenomenon. And, say the sociologists, there are times when the economists seem positively to encourage it. Professor Maynard's recent appearance on a mock-up of a TV game show is cited as a case in point. "How can Williams say a lottery is less rational than QALYs, when at the same time Maynard takes part in a game show where contestants use QALY-type calculations to decide the fate of real-life patients?" asks Dr Pinch. He added "It makes choice by QALY look about as rational as a contestant's choice of a partner on Cilla Black's 'Blind Date'".

Professor Williams seems to have been somewhat more circumspect than his colleague in his use of the media. It is said that he only agrees to appear on radio and TV programmes if he is given some guarantee of editorial control. Williams' appearance on BBC Radio 4's, 'Medicine Now', presented by Jeff Watts, is held up by the health economists as an exemplary case of good publicity. Watts was sympathetic to the QALY concept and the programme, which contained a confrontation between Alan Williams and a critic, the philosopher John Harris, was edited in such a way that Williams easily won the debate.

HEALTH ECONOMISTS REFUSED TREATMENT?

There is increasing concern amongst the York health economists that their involvement with the media has now gone too far. Senior colleagues have apparently expressed worries to Professor Maynard. They stress that although the media have been useful in getting the work of the York Centre better known, their high profile could turn out to be counterproductive. There are even rumours that Maynard's attacks on doctors have led to some York health economists being threatened with withdrawal of medical care.

SOUR GRAPES

But doesn't this concentration on the economists' media involvement smack of sour grapes? Perhaps, deep down, Mulkay and co. feel that they deserve some of the limelight? Vehemently denying anything of the kind, the sociologists argued that their book as a whole demonstrated their concern with much weightier issues.

NO RATIONALE IN RATIONALITY?

The sociologists book is concerned with much more than health economists in the media. The concept of economic rationality itself comes under the microscope. How does the economists' model of the rational individual calculating ends and means measure up when used to recommend changes in the behaviour of complex organizations like the NHS? And what about the economists' stress on the rationality of measurement? The researchers point out that all scientific measures are based upon value choices and assumptions which depend for their credibility upon prevailing scientific opinions. As the history of science shows, these opinions constantly change and will surely change again.

Much of the book is devoted to in-depth technical examinations of the controversial QALY and other measures used by health economists. No QALY-Wallies these sociologists!

ECONOMISTS CHALLENGED TO OPEN DEBATE

Were Mulkay and his group worried about health economists' reactions to their work? "Not really" answered Dr Ashmore.

"We don't expect them to like our book, but we hope we can encourage a fair, rational and open debate." Added Dr Pinch, "If they resist our findings it will be because of their own professional self-interest." In fact the sociologists claim to have experienced resistance already. Professor Williams' response to one of their articles was a robust "So what?" At a recent conference on the inevitable QALY, the sociologists' attempts to introduce the voice of patients into the decision-making process - in the shape of the fictional character, Mrs Jones - was described by Williams as "rubbish." Professor Maynard was for once unavailable for interview. His views on sociology are rumoured to be unpublishable.

ARE SOCIOLOGISTS ANY BETTER?

The York sociologists' research is funded by the same Government body, the Economic and Social Research Council, which funds part of the Centre for Health Economics. Their study is part of a new initiative on science policy. Although the Government may choose to listen to the York sociologists they themselves think it is unlikely and they see their research as much more to do with raising questions rather than presuming to answer them.

But what about sociologists? Can they be any more objective than economists? Mulkay and his colleagues acknowledge the problem. Rather than hiding behind what they see as a spurious objectivity they try and show how their own work is necessarily partial and "only a story." They encourage different readings of their work by telling their story in a variety of ways, some of which are more familiar in the real world of everyday journalism than in the ivory towers of academia.

This last aspect of the York sociologists' work is likely to prove controversial even amongst their sociologist colleagues. When we visited the team we found them surrounded by mounds of broadcast transcripts, press clippings, cardboard and paste. They appeared to be making a collage of health economists' appearances in the media. Dr Ashmore told us "We are trying to compile a fictional press article from all these clippings. Ideally it should tell our analytical story purely by the judicious ordering of the extracts." He told us that he thought of himself as something like a *Sunday Times* "Insight" team reporter investigating health economists and the media. "Our story, like any other story, is bound to be slanted, and hopefully follows the conventions of good journalism. For instance, we have had to quote out of context to achieve the flow." "However", as Dr Pinch insisted, "the main thing is for the story to be interesting. It's certainly been fun to do."

And they call that sociology!

The York Sociology Department study of health economics *Health and Efficiency: A Sociology of Health Economics* is published this week by Open University Press.

5 Measuring the quality of life: a sociological invention

An opening dialogue

You said in Chapter 3 that health economists entered into public debate in order to bring pressure to bear for the implementation of more rational health care policies.

Yes, that's right. My co-authors and I made that claim.

Well, their participation in this debate seems to me to have been an even more dismal failure than their efforts at direct intervention. How on earth can they expect such a blatantly irrational process as that displayed in the preceding chapter to bring about the adoption of rational solutions?

Perhaps they have a more sophisticated appreciation than you of the essentially paradoxical character of the social world. Maybe they realize that irrational commitment is often needed in order to set in motion rational courses of economic action. I know they're not sociologists, but they are probably familiar with Weber's famous argument along these lines in *The Protestant Ethic and the Spirit of Capitalism*.

I'm not sure what you mean by suggesting that the social world is 'essentially paradoxical'. But, whatever you mean, I haven't seen the least sign that health economists would agree with you.

Yes, you're right. I was being excessively charitable. In fact, the economist's entire way of thinking is designed to eliminate such 'unhealthy' phenomena as equivocation, uncertainty, contradiction, ambiguity, paradox and so on. This is particularly evident in the concept of the Quality Adjusted Life Year, or QALY, that featured prominently in the last chapter.

I'm afraid I have to admit that I still don't entirely understand what a QALY is or what it's supposed to do. I think that you should have provided an explanation earlier in the book. That would have helped me, and other readers, to have grasped more clearly what was going on in Chapter 4.

Perhaps. But the reason we didn't explore these technical issues in advance was that the public debate, by its very nature, is supposed to be self-explanatory. Your failure to understand QALYs and other techniques of health economics from the versions given in the media, perhaps suggests that health economists' participation in public debate has been less than successful.

But can you help me come to terms with QALYs? I want to understand this idea in particular because health economists seem to regard it as a major advance.

Well, I'll do my best. You will remember that in Chapter 3 my colleagues and I argued that health economists work with an individualistic model of economic choice and that they try to apply this model to the collective decisions of the NHS?

Er, yes. I have a vague recollection of something like that.

Good. Well, QALYs are thought by many health economists to be a great step forward because they seem to provide, for the first time, a technique for measuring and comparing the various medical benefits produced by the NHS in much the same way that an individual might assess her relative preference for, say avocadoes as compared to oranges.

I'm sorry, but this is getting too complicated. I'm not an economist and I find it difficult to follow. Can we go back to basics?

OK. I hope you will forgive me if my delivery becomes a little didactic. Let's approach the problem by looking closely at a recent paper published by Professor Alan Williams of the University of York. The paper is entitled 'Economics of coronary artery bypass grafting' and appeared in the *British Medical Journal* (vol. 291, 3 August 1985, pp. 326–9). It is this paper which has sparked off the current debate in Britain about QALYs and about economic measurement of the quality of life.

What has 'quality of life' to do with economics or with economists? Surely economics is to do with money and the mechanisms of the market?

Economists would be inclined to treat these comments as simple-minded and as based on a misunderstanding of the nature of their discipline (Culyer 1986). Economics is often said to be the systematic study of all human actions where scarce resources are used to produce valued outcomes (Cooper and Culyer 1973). As your questions imply, people's valuations and the allocation of scarce resources are often mediated through market prices. But this is not always the case. The NHS, for instance, is designed to embody the principle that receipt of medical care shall not depend on the wealth or economic standing of the persons concerned (Williams 1981: 273). Thus, scarce resources are allocated within the NHS to the various forms of medical treatment in order to furnish valued outcomes for patients, but (to some extent) independently of patients' willingness or ability to pay for these treatments. Economists are interested in this kind of provision of valued services precisely *because* the 'normal' market mechanisms are not involved (Williams 1972: 214). In such circumstances, economists are likely to question whether health care can be provided with maximum efficiency when those providing the services are not guided by market forces and to try to identify an effective substitute for market forces (Culyer 1984). To put this in a slightly different way, the NHS constitutes an unusual monopoly in which the producer is not only the sole supplier of goods, but also tells consumers what they need and decides, with little reference to consumers' preferences, what will be produced. In such a situation, economists will try to ensure that the resources available for health care are being used to supply the mixture of services that will produce the most benefit as judged by recipients.

Does this mean that health economists regard themselves as the guardians of patients' interests and that they take their main task to be that of making NHS managers think more carefully about serving those interests?

Although that may be implicit in what health economists say and do, they do not normally depict themselves as directly representing patients. Rather, what they tend to do is to speak as the source of rational courses of action which, if implemented, would work to *everyone's* benefit. It is important to recognize, however, that patients are seldom, if ever, given the opportunity to appraise health economists' proposals for themselves. Because the details of health care policy in Britain are decided formally by NHS managers, but often informally by clinicians, British health economists must approach and persuade both managers and clinicians if they are to influence medical practice. Health economists, however, do not normally seek the approval of patients.

Discussion of the paper begins

In Chapter 2 you showed how health economists catered for the needs of their particular audience. I presume that this is true in the case of Professor Williams.

Yes it is, in several ways. In the first place, the paper is published in a medical journal and is, it would seem, addressed primarily to the members of the health care professions who read such a journal. Second, the paper contains an economic analysis which had previously been presented at a 'consensus development conference on coronary artery bypass surgery' where, it is clear, most of the participants were members of the medical professions. Third, there is a close coincidence between the problem in health care administration which provided the focus for the conference and the problem in economic analysis posed by Williams. Thus in Williams's words, 'the central issue before the conference was whether the number of operations for coronary artery bypass grafting should be increased, decreased, or maintained at its present level' (Williams 1985: 326). The abstract to Williams's own paper begins in almost identical terms: 'To decide whether the number of operations for coronary artery bypass grafting should be increased, maintained at the present level, or decreased we need to know how cost-effective they are relative to other claimants on the resources of the National Health Service' (ibid.: 326).

It appears that Williams's paper is not only addressed to NHS managers, but takes the form of an economic analysis designed to solve the practical problem initially formulated by those managers. When Williams says that 'we' need to know how cost-effective bypass operations are, he speaks both for managers and for economists. In the opening passage of his paper, the discourse of both parties appears to merge in a common search for a solution to a shared problem in the realm of practical action. Although ordinary people are not directly involved in devising this solution, I am sure that Williams would insist that the 'we' of his text also includes the general public, who meet the costs and some of whom may enjoy the benefits.

The next step is presumably to identify the various kinds of constraints which limit managers' and others' actions in order to be able to construct a realistic solution.

Well, no. Williams does not proceed in this way. In his paper, he reformulates the managers' version of their administrative problem in terms of the concepts of health economics, in such a way that it becomes an abstract, idealized problem (see also Williams 1972: 205) to which the answer is obvious once one can discern the relationship between costs and benefits.

> The objective of economic appraisal is to ensure that as much benefit as possible is obtained from the resources devoted to health care. In principle the benefit is measured in terms of the effect on life expectancy adjusted for quality of life. . . . Procedures [medical treatments] should be ranked so that activities that generate more

> gains to health for every £ of resources take priority over those that generate less; thus the general standard of health in the community would be correspondingly higher.
>
> Coronary artery bypass grafting is one of many contenders for additional resources. Ideally, all such contenders should be compared each time a decision on allocation of resources is made to test which should be cut back and which should be expanded.
>
> (Williams 1985: 326)

Although health service managers provide the starting-point for Williams's analysis, their voice quickly disappears from his text and their definitions are quickly replaced by those of the health economist. The practical task of deciding on the allocation of health service resources is transformed by the economist into an exercise in cost–benefit analysis. The course of action required by the health service managers is treated in the course of economic analysis as following necessarily from the balance between costs and benefits as conceived in that analysis. The benefits or outcomes of various forms of medical treatment are defined by the economist in quantifiable terms as the effect on patients' expectation of life with adjustments made for the variable effect on patients' quality of life. Costs are defined, in principle, to include monetary and intangible costs to patients and their families as well as monetary costs to the NHS. But, in practice, only the latter are considered (ibid.: 327). As a result of all this redefinitional work, the economic analysis is able to generate ratios of cost–benefit for various courses of action (medical treatment) and to recommend those actions which furnish the greatest excess of benefit over cost (West 1985/6).

Thus the managers' practical task is reconstituted in the economist's text in such a way that it becomes solvable on the basis of a simple economic metric. This metric generates recommendations because its basic terms carry strong normative weight. No rational actor, it is implied, would incur greater cost than was necessary; nor would s/he refuse additional benefit which was available at no further cost. These assumptions are built into the very meaning of the terms 'cost' and 'benefit'. They are part of the semantics of economic analysis. For instance, if actors chose not to accept what was thought to be additional benefit, it would follow necessarily either that this was in fact not a benefit for them after all or that other aspects of the situation, which had been ignored, constituted benefits or costs in their eyes. This is one reason why the economic metric is immensely powerful and persuasive. Once complex administrative decisions have been reduced to simple, and usually quantified, comparisons of cost and benefit, it comes to seem irrational (or improper, if individuals choose to pursue their private ends rather than the public good) not to act in accordance with the numbers.

You say 'comes to seem irrational'. But surely it is irrational or improper not to obtain the maximum benefit from a given supply of resources. Perhaps the economic metric is persuasive because it does actually solve the managers' problem.

Well, that may be so. Certainly it is the case that Williams is able to conclude his article with a series of strong practical recommendations based on his calculations of costs incurred and quality adjusted life years (QALYs) gained by various forms of medical treatment:

> Resources need to be redeployed at the margin to procedures for which the benefits to patients are high in relation to the costs, such as the insertion of pacemakers for heart block, hip replacement, replacement of valves for aortic stenosis, and coronary artery bypass grafting for severe angina with left main disease and triple vessel disease and moderate angina with left main disease. These treatments should take priority over additional facilities for patients needing kidney transplants and coronary artery bypass grafting for mild angina with left main disease, moderate angina with triple vessel disease or one vessel disease, and severe angina with one vessel disease, for which the costs per quality adjusted life year gained are higher.
>
> (Williams 1985: 329)

But the point I want to stress is that, in the process of providing solutions to the managers' problem, Williams has changed the nature of that problem. He has reformulated the problem in terms of the narrowly conceived discourse of microeconomics. As a result, what might in other discourses be treated as the potential complexities of comparative costs become reduced to single-figure comparisons; and the diverse consequences of specific medical treatments for different groups and individuals become subsumed under aggregate figures representing the 'quality adjusted life years' produced by those treatments. This process of reduction and quantification in terms of concepts with a built-in normative power enables Williams to furnish potent practical proposals. But it also subtly changes the original problem by taking into account only those factors that can be incorporated within the economic metric. For instance, the benefit to be gained from, say, coronary artery surgery *becomes* the number of QALYs it generates and nothing else. The notion of QALYs, however, is furnished by the economists and the procedures for measuring QALYs are devised by economists. Thus, although the economists are, in one sense, adopting the managers' problem and providing a clear, rational solution, they are also, at the same time, redefining and altering the nature of the problem itself. In other words, what begins as the managers' problem is transformed into an economists' problem; and what is eventually offered to the managers, by the economists, is a solution to the economists' analytical problem. A major task facing economists is thus to persuade managers and clinicians that this transformation is actually a revelation of what the problem really is (see Williams 1972: 204). As you will have seen in Chapter 4, they still have some way to go.

Is this meant as a criticism of the economists? Perhaps they might reply that the managers' formulation of the problem had to be abandoned because it was unsolvable in its initial form and that what they have done is to identify the analytical problem that lies behind any practical problem. The fact that the health care professionals were holding a consensus development conference to consider how to allocate resources shows that they were in trouble. How have they dealt with this task in the past?

This is not examined explicitly in Williams's paper. He makes only passing reference to the existing practice of NHS management. He suggests, in particular, that far too much attention has been paid in the past to comparative rates of survival as a criterion for allocating resources to different therapeutic procedures (Williams 1985: 326, 329). This index of medical benefit is misleading, he maintains, because there are many therapies whose main benefit is better quality of life rather then mere prolongation of life at a relatively low level.

However, as we show throughout this book, in other texts by health economists their critique of existing practices of resource allocation in the NHS often goes much further than this. For example, it has been suggested that the NHS suffers from 'the blinkered concerns of cost-minimising accountants and benefit-maximising clinicians' (Maynard 1986: 159), both of which lead to inefficient allocation of resources. In addition, both economists and practitioners recognize that resource allocation is closely linked to political processes within the health service and that resources tend to go, in the idiom of the NHS, to the person or group or specialism that 'shouts the loudest'.

In that case, Williams's proposals are evidently an improvement on existing practices. They replace the irrationalities engendered by the medical status system and by conflict among competing interest groups with a rational calculus designed to link the allocation of resources directly to the overriding goal of the system, namely, the maximization of patients' benefit. Perhaps the appeal of the economists' procedures lies in the fact that they eliminate irrelevant considerations from the decision-making process. What you called above Williams's 'simplification' and 'reduction' of the administrators' complex problem may be more accurately regarded as a clarification of the central issues of resource allocation combined with a procedure for generating appropriate courses of action.

If you were right in suggesting earlier, as it seemed to me, that Williams was imposing the discourse of economics upon the problems of NHS management and replacing their concerns with those of his own discipline, one would surely expect the health service professionals at the conference to respond in a fairly negative manner. Does Williams tell us how they reacted to his supposedly alien discourse?

Williams quotes the following passage from the report of the conference in the second paragraph of his article:

> We were impressed by one method of measurement combining quality and duration of life. Further development of this approach is recommended so that it can be of help not only in comparison between coronary artery bypass surgery and other priorities but also between the various subgroups of patients whom it is proposed should be treated by coronary artery bypass surgery. Such techniques would also help to identify health service estimates which are being continued despite low benefit.
>
> (cited in ibid.: 326)

So they liked it then.

It certainly seems to show that participants at the conference found Williams's procedures and proposals quite persuasive and suggests that the discourse of economics is entering into that of NHS management. However, there may be various reasons for this. In the first place, it may be that the administrators in particular are attracted by the relative simplicity and lack of ambiguity of the economists' decision-making procedures. Such procedures might be favoured, by some parties at least, partly because they make things easier for management. Second, the rhetoric of 'cost', 'benefit' and 'quality of life' is, as I mentioned earlier, difficult to oppose (McCloskey 1985). Thus, if the economists' proposals coincide with certain participants' existing inclinations, they will furnish these participants with a powerful additional weapon in the process of negotiation over the allocation of resources within the NHS. If, for example, you have been pressing for more resources for hip replacements and, by implication, for less resources for costly therapies such as renal dialysis, it will become possible to present your case in more 'objective' terms and to appear to be free from the taint of special pleading. As a result of such considerations, it is likely on most occasions that some participants will have good reason to adopt the proposals generated by the methods of economics (Gabbay 1985/6). But this will not mean that the irrationalities of political negotiation are being replaced by rational economic appraisal. It may simply mean that sections of management and various medical specialisms adopt the procedures and conclusions provided by economists and employ them selectively as a political resource, whilst other equally powerful and numerous people oppose them.

In other words, the sequence may operate like this: The economists take over a practitioners' problem and reformulate it in terms of the economic calculus, thereby generating an economically rational course of action for practitioners. Because all traces of 'special interest' and 'irrationality' have apparently been removed by the economists' procedures, their discourse has a special moral and persuasive power which gives it a peculiar political potency. Economists' proposals, therefore, are welcomed by those participants with whose interests and preconceptions they coincide and are enthusiastically employed by the latter in the course of political negotiation over resource allocation within the NHS. This sets up a strong reaction from those whose interests are harmed. When, as it often does, their opposition to the new procedures focuses on issues of methodology, the very language of political dispute within the NHS begins to absorb and merge with that of economic analysis.

In the course of this process, participants redefine and change the meaning of the solutions to their initial practical problem provided by the economists. If the situation is like this, we have the interestingly paradoxical conclusion that it may be the supposedly non-political or 'scientific' character of the economic calculus which makes it such a powerful political resource for some participants and which generates such strongly negative reactions from others. It may well be that when the economists' recommended solution to the initial problem is brought back into the practical setting, the complexities and 'irrationalities' which were removed for purposes of economic analysis are unavoidably reintroduced and the very meaning of the economists' proposals thereby transformed in their turn.

This is an interesting idea. But it is highly speculative and far removed from both the text with which we began and from the question that I asked.

This is true. However, if we are to understand the practical outcome of Williams's or any other social scientist's efforts to apply their knowledge, we must recognize that any single text operates within a complex series of textual exchanges. Williams can only put his economic expertise to work on behalf of non-economists if he responds to their problems and, in due course, conveys to them effective solutions to those problems. The point I want to emphasize is that important changes of meaning occur as these problems move from one culture or discourse to the other and back again, and that a truly effective 'applied social science' would have to recognize that fact. In the case of health economics, however widely the procedures and formulations furnished by economists may be adopted by participants in the NHS, the meaning of these cultural products and the social uses to which they are put are bound to change within this different social context. If this argument is accepted, it would appear to follow that health economists would be well advised to respond in their analytical procedures and their formal texts to the fact that their rational courses of action can operate fully only within the protected confines of economic discourse.

This argument may sound persuasive within the 'protected confines of sociological discourse', but sociologists are known to be utterly ineffective themselves in the real world of practical action. It seems to me that economists, in contrast, have made very useful contributions in various realms of practical endeavour. In relation to health care, it seems entirely plausible to maintain that economists can often provide better measures than anyone else of the real costs and benefits of practical actions. If this is so, and if health economists can measure patients' quality of life, their intervention will make patients the final arbiter of NHS policy. Economists will be no more than impartial intermediaries. They will certainly be offering NHS managers the products of their own disciplinary culture, but these products will take the form of objective measures of patients' preferences. Thus your remarks about changes of meaning as cultural products move between social contexts are irrelevant. The health economist is not dealing in meanings, but in facts. The ineffectiveness of NHS management in the past has undoubtedly been due to the lack of this kind of factual basis for decision-making. Once the facts about the costs and, particularly, the benefits of various policies become generally available within the NHS, they will severely limit the scope for political manoeuvre and will reveal vested interest, status considerations and other irrationalities for what they really are. I suggest, in opposition to your claims above, that economists' formulations will not be distorted by the culture of the NHS, but that they will provide objective criteria of choice based on patients' experiences which will necessarily bring about major improvements in that culture.

Your faith in the possibility of devising 'objective' measures of quality of life is touching, but I think misplaced. I would argue that the 'facts' generated by *any* group of cognitive experts, whether they are biochemists, radio astronomers or neutrino physicists, should be treated as the cultural products of the respective group and not as re-presentations of phenomena which exist independently of that group and its culture (Pinch 1986). The same argument applies to economists and to other social scientists – including ourselves (Ashmore 1989). Thus when health economists measure the quality of life of patients undergoing different forms of medical treatment, they are not, I suggest, directly identifying what Williams calls 'the benefits to patients' (Williams 1985: 329), but are offering us quantitative indicators of benefits which exist only through the actions and interpretative work of economists, and which are given meaning by economists in the light of their taken-for-granted assumptions about the way that patients, and people in general, experience the world.

I will ignore your provocative remark about my faith in economists being touching and concentrate on your own factual claim regarding the cultural production of facts. Can you show how it applies to health economists and the quality of life?

Measuring the quality of life

In order to do this, I must describe briefly how quality of life is measured. Although economists use various techniques to measure quality of life, I will focus on the procedure used in Williams's 1985 paper, which is designed to specify the variations in QALYs produced by different medical treatments (see also Gudex 1986; Kind, Rosser and Williams 1982; and Rosser and Kind 1978). The first step is to identify those aspects of quality of life that are to be measured. Williams adopts a procedure which deals with physical mobility (or degree of disability) and with level of distress (of which physical pain will be a major component).

Surely there is more to 'quality of life' than this?

Yes, Williams is well aware of that. He acknowledges that the judgements on which his measures are based are 'crude and in need of refinement' (Williams 1985: 326). However, physical mobility and freedom from distress are fundamental aspects of our life experience in the sense that without them we are unable 'to perform the activities of daily living and to engage in normal social interaction' (ibid.: 326). When we are physically confined and in pain or otherwise distressed, we are prevented from enjoying even the commonplace pleasures of everyday life, let alone the more subtle aspects of high-quality living.

That seems reasonable. But how can you measure physical mobility and distress? I suppose there must be physiological indicators of the level of pain; and I suppose you could fit pedometers to sick and healthy people and compare how far they walk each day. But distress seems more nebulous than pain, and I wonder whether you can combine such different measures of such different phenomena into a single index of quality of life.

Well, neither Williams nor other health economists choose those kinds of physical indicators. They adopt what Williams calls elsewhere a 'feeling-functional' measure (Williams 1981: 273). What this means, I think, is that he is trying to measure how people subjectively experience and evaluate various states of disability and distress in relation to their normal patterns of life. He is attempting to assess in quantitative terms people's feelings about and preferences for various physical conditions which are below their normal quality of life.

So QALYs provide a measure of what one might call negative preferences. They tell us how far people dislike certain unpleasant states. Is that right?

That's correct. I think QALYs could, perhaps, have been more accurately called LYSPAMs, that is, 'life years spent in pain and misery'. But that rather unattractive acronym might not have captured economists' or administrators' imaginations so effectively or aroused so much controversy in the media. However, whatever we call it, this negative indicator seems appropriate when the analyst is trying to measure the outcomes of medical treatments which are intended, as far as possible, to return patients to normal health. The indicator used by Williams, therefore, takes normal health as its bench-mark and measures how far various conditions are judged by ordinary people to fall below that level.

But I still don't understand how this rather intangible negative utility is to be measured.

The procedure is as follows. First, allocate a value of 1 to the state of normal health and 0 to the state of death. Second, specify a series of intermediate states involving different degrees and combinations of disability and distress. The measure employed by Williams makes use of eight conditions of disability, ranging from 'no disability' through 'severe social disability' and 'unable to undertake any paid employment' to 'unconscious'. These are then combined with four levels of distress – namely none, mild, moderate and severe – to give a quality of life (disability and distress) matrix with twenty-nine possible conditions. The third step is to select a sample of respondents[1] and to obtain from them numerical scores up to a score of 1 for each of the twenty-nine conditions. The scores of individual respondents are then aggregated to form quantitative measures of the sample's, and indirectly the community's, valuation of the quality of life associated with various states of health (Williams 1981: 276). The values given by Williams decline in a fairly straightforward manner as the degree of disability and the level of distress increase. The findings confirm that there are few people who prefer to be in a state of extreme distress or who place a high value on being confined to a wheelchair or lying unconscious in bed. (See note 1 at the end of this chapter for the actual figures.)

If these are the results, is this rather complex exercise informative? And is it of any use?

I don't think it is *very* informative in itself, although we may find it interesting that some conditions seem to be widely regarded as worse than death; for example, being confined to bed in a state of severe distress gets a score of −1.486. However, the quality of life matrix certainly is useful; at least, many health economists maintain that it is and health care managers are beginning to agree. From the economists' perspective it doesn't matter that the ranking of states of health seems pretty obvious. Indeed, they might reasonably claim that this is a sign of the validity of their procedures. The critical point is, for economists, that they now have a quantified index of people's judgements of the quality of life associated with typical states of health. This means that we no longer have to make unreliable qualitative estimates of whether, say, hip replacements do more good than coronary artery bypass grafting. We can now quantify the benefit gained from radically different therapies using a common unit of value and, what is more, we can fairly easily work out how much each unit of value (QALY) costs in different areas of medicine and, therefore, where we can get best value for money.

I understand the general argument. But I still don't quite understand how you get from Williams's quality of life matrix to the measurement of quality adjusted life years.

In order to do this, you need some more information from patients and/or doctors. Basically, you require a profile of what happens to a typical patient over time after a specific medical treatment has occurred. In Williams's paper, doctors provide this information. But, in due course, patients will probably be employed to provide more accurate data. However they are obtained, the analyst's task is to interpret these profiles in terms of the aggregate quality of life scores attached to the various states of health identified in the matrix. For example, if a typical patient has an additional life expectancy of three years after having operation X and the matrix scores for those three years are 0.5, 0.3 and 0.2, the typical benefit of that operation will be 1.0 QALY (0.5 + 0.3 + 0.2). Operation Y, in contrast, may add ten years to a patient's life expectancy with a quality of life score of 0.9 throughout. The QALY for operation Y, therefore, is 9 (0.9 × 10), and we can conclude that operation Y is nine times more valuable than operation X.

QALYs do seem to be very useful. By turning people's subjective judgements into an objective index, obtained by means of systematic and explicit procedures, they seem to help us to make rational choices. In the hypothetical example that you gave, we would clearly choose to divert resources from X to Y until their benefits were equal at the margin. You see, I'm not entirely ignorant of economics.

Well, a little economics is a dangerous thing. You've forgotten to consider costs. One of the great advantages of QALYs is that they enable us to compute a single-figure ratio in which benefit gained is related to cost incurred. Thus, if operation X cost £100 and operation Y £900, the cost for each additional quality adjusted life year would be identical and nothing at all would be gained by altering things. However, in general terms, once costs have been taken into account, we can use QALYs to construct a 'league table' of medical treatments which will show clearly where resources can be redeployed to provide greater benefit for patients in their own terms. Williams begins to do this in his paper. Thus the QALY can be regarded as a technique devised by economists to solve administrators' problems of resource allocation in such a way that patients derive the maximum benefit from doctors' actions.

That sounds wonderful. No doubt there will be many practical difficulties to be overcome. But by making people's preferences available to NHS managers and clinicians in quantitative form, the health economists do seem to be helping to construct a system of health care in which the patient's welfare or quality of life becomes the primary focus at last.

I'm not willing to accept that formulation without amendment. I would say that they are trying to construct a system in which the patient's welfare or quality of life *as seen by (some) health economists* is the primary focus.

Isn't that splitting hairs? You're quibbling over my choice of words. The fact is that the economists are going to patients, or at least to people who are potential patients, and obtaining the preferences that they carry about in their heads. In this basic respect, therefore, it is patients who will, ultimately, determine health care policy; that is, if the health economists' proposals are put into effect. However, I expect you will object to this interpretation on the grounds that the economists' recommendations will be changed, as you argued earlier, by the administrators and by political negotiation within the NHS.

Further implications are explored

No, I don't want to repeat that point. I want to concentrate now on the relationship between the economist and the *patient*. I'm very doubtful about your claim, which I think is Williams's claim as well, that the health economists' measurement techniques correctly represent patients' preferences. For instance, when we examine his paper we see that whereas health administrators *do* contribute actively to that paper in that the provide the initial problem and they are given space in which to express their support for further development of his investigations, patients never appear actively in the text at all. Generalizations about patients' inclinations are sometimes offered by the author; for example, that 'some patients are willing to sacrifice a measure of life expectancy for a better quality of life' (Williams 1985: 326). But the textual voice on such occasions is always that of the economist. We are never given direct access to the reasoning practices of patients or ordinary people in relation to the issues as they might define them. This is very clear in the case of people's judgements of quality of life and the indices of quality adjusted life years. This material is always presented in tabular or graphical form. Consequently, in this text, we are never concerned with any individual person's actual evaluations but with aggregate evaluations prepared by economists or by their colleagues. It is quite misleading, therefore, to suggest that QALYs can bring the preferences of the general public directly to bear upon health care policy. What QALYs may do is to introduce into the policy arena some consideration of responses obtained from ordinary people. But these responses are given meaning by and processed in aggregate terms by economic experts.

But surely this is standard procedure in the social sciences. Would you prefer Williams to write chatty biographies about what Mrs Jones thinks and then generalize from Mrs Jones to the world at large? The use of aggregate measures is simply, if I may use the word in this context, an 'economical' way of expressing a central tendency within the group. If Williams did not aggregate his data, we would be lost in a welter of discrepant individual judgements and quite unable to come to any conclusion about what should be done to improve NHS policy. By means of aggregation, however, he can convey communal judgements with precision and make possible a rational choice of outcomes in accordance with those judgements.

I agree that this is normal procedure for much quantitative social science and that, within this approach, the range of methodological alternatives is strictly limited. The point I want to emphasize, however, is that such research methods do not represent the judgements of individual respondents, but rather create a new reality out of those judgements. Moreover, this analyst's reality can come to be regarded as 'more real' than that of the individuals it is supposed to represent. In the case of quality of life measures, for instance, as Williams notes in an earlier paper, the value that 'emerges may not coincide with the actual valuations of any particular individual' (Williams 1981: 277). Yet it is the value produced by the expert and given meaning in terms of the expert's analytical assumptions which is to be used as the basis for policy and as a guide for practical action. In this case, it is the economist alone who is allowed to speak on behalf of potential patients as a collectivity, even though no individual members of the collectivity may endorse the values proposed by the economist. It is accepted, of course, that the potential patient can give a true account of his or her personal preferences. But the precise measurement of the preferences of the group can be provided only by the economist. Indeed, if the valuations that emerged actually coincided with those of any particular individual or group of individuals, this could be taken as grounds for suggesting that the measurements were defective. (These points apply equally to any sociologist or other social scientist trying to measure group phenomena.) This is what I meant when I suggested earlier that the facts about quality of life furnished in Williams's text, and used as the basis for practical recommendations, are not patients' facts but economists' facts. They exist only through the actions and interpretative work carried out by economists. They are, therefore, resistant to challenge by potential patients, as are the practical recommendations to which they give rise, unless patients adopt the economists' basic assumptions about the possibility of aggregating individual preferences.

But this is only because social scientists have a unique ability to identify and give voice to patients' preferences. Their findings and eventual recommendations are severely restricted by the facts of the matter. Economists, for example, do not invent these preferences. What they do is to use their special knowledge and techniques to reveal preferences which already exist out there in the real world. In other words, economists are constrained by the data. Their measurements and conclusions, although they may not and perhaps should not coincide exactly with those of individual patients, do genuinely represent the average of the judgements of the group in question. It is true that we cannot know the nature of this collective judgement without economists' (or some other social scientists') help, but the reality which they make available to us is not their *reality. It is that of the community of people from whom their data are obtained.*

Perhaps. But this view depends on the assumption that the 'data' which supposedly 'constrain' economists are not their own creation and that they do not impose their own meanings on those data. I think that both these assumptions are wrong. Shall I explain why?

Please do.

In an earlier paper to which I have referred several times, Williams (1981) lists a series of six conditions which have to be satisfied when individuals express their evaluations of the quality of life associated with specific states of health. He states there that the analyst must try to ensure that respondents think of each health state as existing for the same length of time, that they judge each state on the basis of its intrinsic 'enjoyability', that all states are evaluated as if the respondent were in them now, that no element of prognosis 'seeps in', and so on. These conditions, he comments, are 'very stringent' and they 'make empirical work to elicit such evaluations rather difficult' (Williams 1981: 275).

Clearly, the analyst can try to make sure, as far as possible, that these conditions are satisfied by formulating questions in an appropriate manner. But it is impossible to tell from respondents' evaluations themselves, that is from the 'raw data', whether or not judgements have been carried out in the ideal fashion required by the measurement technique. What happens in practice, of course, is that analysts simply interpret the data on the assumption that these conditions have been met. Thus in his short 1985 paper in the *British Medical Journal* Williams makes no mention of these stringent methodological requirements. In this text, respondents' quality of life scores are treated as unproblematic in the sense that the background assumptions on which their analytical meaning, and their practical implications, depend are left implicit. As a result, the ever-present possibility, in principle, of alternative interpretations becomes hidden from view.

If we worry about the 'ever-present possibility of alternative interpretations' we will never solve our analytical problems; nor will our research produce results which are useful in the practical world. This kind of constant concern with interpretative uncertainties seems to be one of the major differences between sociologists and economists. Sociologists sit there contemplating their own navels, or in this case someone else's epistemological difficulties, whilst economists get on with the real job of solving problems and improving our understanding (Thunhurst 1985/6). In Williams's case, you mentioned earlier that he admits that his present data are crude. Presumably this implies a recognition on his part that he has had to make assumptions in order to interpret the data. But these assumptions can be checked in future studies and the conclusions made increasingly rigorous.

That may be so. But it seems to me that many of these assumptions become taken utterly for granted and, consequently, are never put to the test. For example, in Williams's 1985 paper he notes that the evaluations of the doctors in the sample of respondents who provided the quality of life scores tended to differ significantly from those of the rest of the sample. In particular, the doctors tended to give lower scores than did other people. Williams concludes that these doctors 'appeared to have a much greater aversion to disability and distress than the population at large' and that they therefore overvalued 'reductions in disability and distress compared with the rest of the population' (Williams 1985: 327).

In reaching this conclusion, Williams has assumed that there are no relevant variations within the sample in respondents' ability to understand the quality of life measure and to comply with the stringent conditions which it requires. In other words, he seems at this early stage to have forgotten that the meaning given to respondents' scores depends on certain assumptions about how the scores were produced. As a result, he has not considered the possibility that systematic differences within the sample may well be due to differences in respondents' understanding of the measurement procedure. It seems just as reasonable to assume, however, that doctors, due to their high level of training in relation to issues of health care, are more able than the other members of the sample to make the precise and subtle assessments required by the quality of life measure. But if we make this assumption, we will be led to conclude that the average scores for the sample as a whole are inaccurate and that the scores furnished by the sub-sample of doctors may be a more valid indicator of quality of life valuations for the population at large. Thus Williams ignores the possibility that the stringent conditions required in this line of research may be satisfied to varying degrees by different kinds of respondent and infers that the different responses of doctors and others indicate genuine evaluative differentials. In contrast, my alternative interpretation assumes that doctors may understand the nature and requirements of the measuring device better than other people and that their scores are more accurate and furnish a better guide for practical action.

I am not trying to insist that this alternative interpretation is the correct one and that Williams is necessarily mistaken. The main point I wish to make is that Williams's data alone do not determine his conclusions about quality of life or about practical action. I have tried to show that, by varying our background assumptions, we can derive significantly different conclusions from the same set of quantitative scores; and that entirely reasonable alternative assumptions are available. I suggest, therefore, that, if we wish to understand how Williams's conclusions about QALYs and medical treatments are produced, we must concentrate not on his data but on the assumptions which are used to give meaning to those data.

Are you suggesting that there are further assumptions relevant to QALYs which are not identified in Williams's earlier (1981) paper?

Yes, I think there are (see Strong 1985/6; Gabbay 1985/6). The assumptions formulated in Williams's 1981 paper are relatively specific and closely linked to quality of life measures. But there are other presuppositions evident in his work that are probably basic to much economic analysis. I don't want to overwhelm you with a lengthy disquisition on the nature of economic discourse (see McCloskey 1985). Instead, I will just comment briefly on three important background assumptions. I shall call them the assumptions of correspondence, stability and quantification. I will argue that these assumptions, although taken for granted in, for example, Williams's text, are open to question.

The first assumption is that the categories used by the analyst correspond with or capture the evaluations that respondents make in the course of ordinary everyday life. Unless this assumption is made, the analyst can hardly use her or his findings to recommend changes in NHS practice. Yet it seems a highly unlikely assumption because the analyst's categories are so abstract and artificial, because the judgements of quality of life elicited by the research technique are so far removed from those which occur in real social situations, and because the analysts state that their measurements actually change respondents' evaluations. For instance, the scores used in Williams's paper are generated by presenting to respondents a prearranged set of categories of disability and distress, clearly ranked in terms of severity, and by asking respondents to allocate numerical estimates of quality of life to these abstract conditions. It is hardly surprising that such a procedure generates a smooth distribution of aggregate values. But are these values in any way related to people's everyday judgements or are they a predictable response to an abstractly conceived measurement technique?

It is clear that in everyday life people are not required to distinguish between carefully defined categories, but to choose between ill-defined courses of action in situations which are complex, diffuse and subject to change (West 1985/6). Judgements of quality of life, I suggest, may well be made quite differently in these two radically different kinds of context. Indeed, Williams recognizes this, at least implicitly, when he discusses the stringent conditions of measurement which make empirical research in this area so difficult. In ordinary life, the experimental conditions identified by Williams as being required by the measurement procedure are never satisfied. It seems to me, therefore, rather difficult to assume that the scores elicited by the abstract, artificial measurement technique correspond in any straightforward way to the judgements that people make in normal circumstances.

The assumption of correspondence seems to become even more doubtful when one reads another previous paper which maintains that the subjects involved in evaluating the states of ill-health according to this procedure 'experienced the interview as traumatic and felt that it changed their perception of illness' (Kind, Rosser and Williams 1982: 167). If the scores obtained from respondents do express perceptions that have been altered by the act of measurement, it seems clear that these scores cannot correspond with or properly represent the values of a larger population whose members have not undergone measurement and whose normal procedures of evaluation seem to be so different from those used in the measurement device that the latter are experienced as profoundly disturbing.

At the very least, I suggest, we have to conclude that social scientists measuring quality of life in this way are assuming a correspondence between their measurements and people's ordinary judgements that is rather doubtful. Although the correspondence between social scientists' observations and the values of the population at large is far from certain, it is none the less taken for granted in the course of analysis. It is an assumption that is routinely brought to the data by the analyst and is used to give meaning to the data and to project that meaning upon the wider social world with which s/he is ultimately concerned.

The other two assumptions that I mentioned before operate, I think, in much the same way. The assumption of stability presupposes that people carry around a set of internal preferences or evaluations which are relatively stable. Given this assumption, the task of the researcher is to elicit and record those individual, internal states as precisely as possible. However, there is now a large body of research showing that the values forthcoming from particular respondents change significantly in accordance with variations in the process of elicitation and also that there appears to be little relationship between the values thus elicited and the choices actors make in real situations (Denzin 1970, Part 4; Denzin 1978). It may be, therefore, that we should treat participants' evaluations as variable *social* phenomena and their evaluative responses, not as expressions of stable underlying preferences, but as reactions to socially defined situations (Cicourel 1964). In so far as we come to recognize the social character of the research process and the socially generated character of subjects' responses, the assumption that the social researcher is eliciting relatively stable and context-free evaluations becomes much less plausible. Once again, we come to see the assumption of stability as a presupposition which is taken for granted when the analyst treats his or her measurements as referring to stable preferences which exist independently of the process of measurement.

Similarly, the assumption of quantification seems to me to be quite unrealistic. It is fundamental to the procedure for constructing QALYs that respondents are required to make precise numerical assessments of the conditions provided by the analyst. Unless this is done, the benefits of different treatments cannot be measured and cost–benefit ratios cannot be derived. The analysis seems to assume, therefore, that the numbers assigned by respondents have some real meaning for them in ordinary situations and that these numbers express quantifications that are already implicit in individual respondents' scales of preference. We have to accept, of course, that analysts can persuade many respondents to assign numbers to the abstract categories which they provide, even though this process may often be experienced as traumatic. But we know from other studies that subjects in the experimental context can also be persuaded to pass what are taken to be damaging charges of electricity through innocent people (Milgram 1963, 1974). In other words, there may be good grounds for doubting whether actions such as quantification that are accomplished in the research setting closely reflect the processes which normally occur in everyday situations. Given the wholly artificial nature of the measurement procedure, it seems likely that the smooth distribution of scores produced in these attempts to measure quality of life is a result of respondents' recognition of a quantification already implicit in the analyst's prearranged categories.

You're arguing, then, that people's everyday judgements of quality of life are not quantitative, are not stable and do not correspond with the analyst's abstract categories.

Conclusions are drawn concerning social science and practical action

I'm arguing that the analyst, in using certain kinds of measurement techniques and in interpreting results in a particular manner, is making *assumptions* on these issues and that entirely reasonable alternative assumptions are possible. I'm also arguing that quality of life measures and QALYs are not re-presentations of people's pre-existing values. They are, I suggest, the interpretative outcome of a special, and indeed rather peculiar, form of social interaction between economists and ordinary people. Although QALYs are presented as an accurate reflection of the latter's preferences, ordinary people are only able to express their preferences through a measurement procedure which is constructed in terms of social scientists' preconceptions. Potential patients contribute only indirectly to economists' accounts of their preferences, and it is economists who establish the *meaning* of that contribution.

To return to what I was saying earlier, economists use their results to speak on behalf of patients and to specify what actions would best serve patients' interests. Yet economists' results and recommendations depend on the background assumptions of their disciplinary culture. If that culture were different, what economists say on our behalf would be different. It is in this sense that the facts expressed in QALYs are not patients' facts, but economists' facts.

I accept much of what you have said about the interpretative dominance of the economist over his or her subjects of study. But in this respect, economics is surely no different from other social sciences; except perhaps that economists have used this dominance to greater scientific effect than, say, sociologists, who have been excessively concerned with the limitations of their own findings.

It's true that economists have been relatively successful in shaping the factual world of economic phenomena in accordance with the assumptions of their own disciplinary culture. Unlike sociologists, economists have more or less consciously adopted the simplest possible model of the social actor (namely, a maximizer of utility) and have used it to generate a wide range of rigorous, elegant analyses (Culyer 1984). They have also begun to devise ways of treating complex social processes, like systems for delivering health care, in terms of this simplistic model of the individual actor undertaking rational choices. For example, as I said at the beginning of this discussion, the QALY succeeds in making our collective choice between, say, hip replacements and renal dialysis, appear to be as straightforward and obvious as an individual shopper's choice between avocadoes and oranges. In this respect, simplification and quantification have paid off analytically; and if economists' claims were confined to their professional journals, the adequacy of their analyses would be for them to decide. However, when economists intervene in the realm of practical action, their analytical concern with a world of idealized economic phenomena and, in particular, their failure to recognize the social character of the research process and the social character of their own knowledge claims, may become significant for outsiders like ourselves.

You mean because economists imply that they know, or that they will know in due course, our real preferences and that they are, therefore, speaking and acting on our behalf, whether we realize it or not.

Yes, that's right. We need to understand economists' discourse because it often appears textually to be a re-presentation of the general public's preferences and as such, as I suggested earlier, it may be absorbed into the decision-making practices of the NHS and used there as a basis for action and/or as a potent source of legitimation. It's important to remember that the range of potential application of concepts such as the 'QALY' is very wide indeed. Given that economics is taken to be 'the systematic study of all human actions where scarce resources are used to produce valued outcomes', we can expect that, given the opportunity, economists will speak on our behalf in almost any area of practical activity.

You seem determined to find fault with the health economists. They are simply trying to use their distinctive skills to help other people. And all you can do is to criticize.

What I have to say must appear to be critical because it's my task as a sociologist to refuse to accept the taken-for-granted assumptions of those I study and to make them available for inspection (Schutz 1972). But I may have another unacknowledged reason for criticizing the health economists (see Strong 1979). It may be that I have to prove them to be wrong, if I am to be able to establish the analytical and/or practical value of my own contribution. I think that there is an important general point here about using one's knowledge to assist others; namely, in order to be of assistance one's knowledge must be shown to differ significantly from and to be rather better than that of the recipient.

That seems a rather trivial observation to me.

Perhaps it is. But the need to distinguish one's knowledge from the recipient's can have major consequences for the social negotiation of knowledge. There's a good example of this in relation to QALYs. Williams argues, you will remember, that in judging the success of medical treatments administrators and others have relied unduly in the past on measuring improvements in patients' life expectancy. He suggests that this is quite unsatisfactory for the considerable number of treatments whose main effect is on quality of life rather than the duration of life. It is for this reason that Williams's measure of medical effectiveness, the QALY, combines life expectancy with quality of life in a single indicator. However, in the matrix of scores for quality of life used by Williams, the range of variation tends to be rather narrow. More specifically, eighteen out of the twenty-nine scores are between 0.9 and 1.0. As I explained earlier, Williams's quality of life scores measure how far various states of health are judged to fall below a normal quality of life. The figures in the matrix therefore suggest, if one adopts Williams's interpretation that they accurately represent respondents' ordinary judgements, that in the majority of conditions (eighteen out of twenty-nine) quality of life is deemed to be almost indistinguishable from normal. A condition would have to involve confinement to a wheelchair or something of that kind before respondents in the sample used by Williams begin to judge the quality of life as falling below 90 per cent of normal. One consequence of this small range of variation is that quality of life scores tend to make a relatively minor contribution to Williams's QALYs; variations in life expectancy contribute much more to the final indicator and to the supposed differences in the benefits produced by various medical treatments.

This, of course, somewhat weakens the argument for the superiority of the QALY over the administrators' customary indicator of life expectancy. It also means that the QALYs generated using Williams's quality of life matrix may in many cases furnish little additional information for the policy-makers in the NHS. However, since the publication of Williams's paper in 1985 this problem has been noted by other health economists, and moves have been made to ensure that, in the next generation of quantitative measures, the scores for quality of life will vary over a wider range (Drummond 1986; Gudex 1986). I have no doubt that a wide spread of quality of life scores will become a standard feature of QALYs in due course and that measures such as Williams's will be regarded as crude and defective preliminary attempts. Williams himself prepares the way for this when he stresses that his data are undoubtedly 'in need of refinement' (Williams 1985: 326).

Clearly, from the point of view of the health economists working on QALYs, they are engaged here in devising better indicators (Williams 1972: 204). But, from the point of view of an outsider like myself, they also appear to be engaged in distinguishing their product and their knowledge from that already available to the NHS administrators. There seems to me to be no particular reason to assume that people's real judgements of quality of life must involve a wide range of values rather than a narrow spread. As I mentioned earlier, Williams rejects doctors' scores as atypical because they have a wider spread than those produced by the rest of the sample. Moreover, we can have no independent indicator of these judgements which would help us to decide either way. It seems to me, therefore, that the wide range of values now being built into the measuring devices is not an observable feature of ordinary people's assessments of quality of life. It is, rather, a result of health economists' presupposition that there is some quantifiable phenomenon out there called 'evaluation of quality of life' which formerly was inaccessible to administrators, combined with health economists' commitment to measuring this phenomenon in a way which will enable them to make a distinctive contribution to the administrative process. In my view, contrary to the impression conveyed by the scientific discourse of measurement used by economists, quality of life is not a measurable phenomenon out there in the social world, but an interpretative by-product of the social interaction between ordinary people, doctors, NHS managers and, most important of all in this context, health economists.

There you go being critical again. One thing that worries me is that you don't seem to apply your own kind of critique to yourself. Your research is as much a social act as the economists' and as much a process of attributing meaning guided by assumptions current within your discipline. Why should I accept the points that you have made against health economics if you avoid applying them to your own assertions?

It's entirely up to you. You can accept my arguments if you find them persuasive and reject them if you do not, but obviously I hope to persuade you. Anyway, I don't see my arguments as being directed particularly against health economics or health economists. My general claims about the social production and application of knowledge would indeed apply to any field of intellectual endeavour, including my own. What I've been trying to do, analytically, is to draw attention to some of the specific background assumptions which form part of the social practice of health economics and to the conventional nature of the textual forms used by economists, as well as by most other social scientists, whereby the contingent, socially generated claims of specific groups of 'knowledge producers' come to be depicted as, and sometimes mistaken for, the preferences of the population at large or the 'real world' of everyday action. At the same time, I have a practical message. I'm saying to anyone who is willing to listen to me, 'Be careful. This is only one way of looking at the world. There can be other versions of the facts and other rational and practically effective courses of action.'

So that's your version of the facts?

It is. But I have tried not to hide the partiality of my account behind the language of measurement and the supposedly universal discourse of scientific fact. I make no claims for any privileged position and it is for you to decide on these matters for yourself.

Well, I'm rather disappointed if that's all you have to say. I am obliged to point out that you have engaged in a form of intellectual cheating. By making such strong criticisms of health economists you have implied that better procedures could be devised and put to work. But then you let yourself off the hook by admitting at the end that the same points could probably be made about anything. You've led me on, encouraging me to expect that you are going to provide a practical solution of your own – and now you've welshed on the deal. I would go so far as to allege that your moral condemnation of health economists has boomeranged, revealing the moral culpability of your own position.

I'm very sorry that you feel like that. It hadn't occurred to me that you would expect me to step into the health economists' shoes. I have to say that I refuse to replace their analytical expertise with my own. I did not invite you into my text in order to convince you that I and my sociological colleagues can provide better practical advice in the realm of health care than those academics in the next department. In fact, I am not offering to use my analytical expertise to help *you*. On the contrary, I have been trying to clarify these misunderstandings as a prelude to asking you to help *me*. Before I can hope to do anything of practical benefit, I need to find some way of bringing your voice, the questioning voice of the potential recipient, more actively into my texts. Unless I can engage you in true dialogue, applied sociological analysis, however well intentioned, will remain like that of the health economists, a discourse of domination. But are you willing to help?

I can't decide at the moment. The economists seem more like real experts to me. They have got definite policies based on measurements of the public's preferences. I am attracted by your offer to take an active part in the analysis, but in order to make up my mind I would very much like to hear what Professor Williams himself has to say about our discussion. Is that possible?

Yes, if you insist. It so happens that there is a published response from Alan Williams to an earlier version of this chapter (Mulkay *et al.* 1987). If you feel that it will be helpful, you can read his reply below.

Measuring quality of life: a comment by Alan Williams

Scientific analysis requires simplification and abstraction. It entails associating selected 'real world' phenomena with particular concepts in a theoretical model. The logic of the model itself should have been thoroughly explored, so that the properties of its individual elements, their interrelationships and their implications will be well understood in the abstract. These general properties, interrelationships and implications are then worked through as if applicable to the particular selected 'real world' phenomena, and are then interpreted back from the abstractions of the model to refer to their supposed counterparts in the phenomena of the real world.

Those statements are true of scientific analysis in general, so since economists' analyses purport to be scientific analyses they are true of economists' analyses too.

That seems to be the essence of what Mulkay *et al.* are saying in their rather wordy, contrived dialogue, and if that is indeed their message it is unexceptionable, but unoriginal, and my remaining disagreements with them can be regarded as mere matters of detail. Among these matters of detail are the contradictory passages which seem to argue, on the one hand, that the specific data used on people's preferences are highly suspect and probably inaccurate (because they change so little over wide ranges of disability and distress) and, on the other hand, their initial dismissal of these same data as uninformative because they tell us exactly what we would expect. Catch 23? There also seem to be some inconclusive comments concerning the appropriate way to convert individuals' values into group values. I have tried to be explicit in my writings on QALYs that aggregation is not simply a technical matter, but a process involving important ethical assumptions, e.g. that adding different people's QALYs together implies that one year of healthy life expectancy is regarded as of equal value to everybody, and that being dead is equally bad for everybody. The QALY approach does not depend on those particular assumptions, and if other ethical assumptions about distributive justice were thought to be more appropriate other methods of aggregation would be appropriate.

The advantage of a systematic and explicit analytical model is that you can see where you are with it, and it is interesting to note how much of their 'sociological' critique of QALYs depends on methodological points which have already been made by economists themselves concerning the limitations of their own work. Indeed, I see little that is particularly 'sociological', and much that is generally methodological, in their critique. Moreover, it is not clear what the economists' approach is being compared with. What is the gold standard here? How do alternative approaches stand up to the tests that are being applied?

This brings me to the one point of substance on which I think Mulkay *et al.* are weak. Had I continued the first paragraph of this comment at the same level of generality with which I began, the next couple of sentences would have run thus:

A 'good' analytical model is one which simplifies away inessentials, and offers useful insights by clear and appropriate interpretation of its results. A 'bad' analytical model is one which simplifies away essentials and/or misleads by misinterpreting the 'real-world' implications of the results.

Again, these statements are true of scientific analysis in general and, to the extent that economic analysis purports to be scientific analysis, are true of economic analysis in particular.

But who is to judge whether a piece of analysis is good or bad? If it is purely 'explanatory' the classic test is its predictive (or postdictive) power compared with its rivals. But if, as in this case, it is normative (i.e. offers advice to someone on how best to behave) then the test must instead be (a) whether the objectives assumed in the model are indeed the objectives of the persons to whom the advice is addressed, and (b) whether the advice, if followed, does in fact lead to better outcomes for those persons than following other advice. Both of these are matters of fact to be tested empirically, and we can only wait and see how QALYs will fare.

But Mulkay *et al.* seem determined that QALYs shall not win *whatever* the outcome! If, say, NHS managers rejected our results, that is taken to indicate failure on our part. But if they accept and act on our results (and are happy with the outcome) 'it may simply mean that sections of management and various medical specialisms adopt the procedures and conclusions provided by economists and employ them selectively as a political resource, whilst other equally powerful and numerous people oppose them'. Catch 24?

My own credo in this matter is that it is the task of all applied social scientists to attempt to formulate, as systematically as possible, the processes of thought and discussion which precede decisions, and to help the people involved to gather and deploy all the information they can that bears on those decisions, in a manner that makes sense to the people involved. All such information will always be incomplete and will never be wholly reliable, so the pragmatic test is: is it better than anything else on offer at present? And for us in the research business, the next question is: what can we do now to ensure that we shall be able to do even better in future? I am confident that we do have something valuable (though not perfect) to offer *right now*, and that we shall have something even better (though still not perfect) to offer in the future. But however good we get to be at our respective tasks, the statements in my opening paragraph will still be true! So what?

(Williams 1987)

Note

1. The sample consisted of seventy subjects with the following range of backgrounds: ten patients from medical wards, ten psychiatric in-patients, ten experienced state registered general nurses, ten experienced state registered psychiatric nurses, ten doctors each with a Membership or Fellowship of at least one Royal College and twenty healthy volunteers (see Rosser and Kind 1978; Kind, Rosser and Williams 1982; Gudex 1986). According to one insider/commentator 'this base of seventy subjects should be much larger and wider . . . to ensure that the valuations used are not skewed by any bias within the group of subjects, and . . . are representative for the general population' (Gudex 1986: 18). The fact that this original sample is generally understood to be 'technically inadequate' does not, we think, affect *our* critique. Were the sampling procedures and the subsequent scales to be improved, as most people involved in research on QALYs would wish them to be, the measurements would still be based on the assumptions of correspondence, stability and quantification.

The following tables on p. 114 detail the classification of illness states and the matrix of evaluations of the original sample of respondents.

Table 5.1 The classification of illness states

Disability		*Distress*	
I	No disability	A	No distress
II	Slight social disability	B	Mild
III	Severe social disability and/or slight impairment of performance at work Able to do all housework except very heavy tasks	C	Moderate
		D	Severe
IV	Choice of work or performance at work very severely limited Housewives and old people able to do light housework only but able to go out shopping		
V	Unable to undertake any paid employment Unable to continue any education Old people confined to home except for escorted outings and short walks and unable to do shopping Housewives able only to perform a few simple tasks		
VI	Confined to chair or to wheelchair or able to move around in the house only with support from an assistant		
VII	Confined to bed		
VIII	Unconscious		

Table 5.2 The valuation matrix as scored by the original seventy respondents

Disability rating	*Distress rating*			
	A	B	C	D
I	1.000	0.995	0.990	0.967
II	0.990	0.986	0.973	0.932
III	0.980	0.972	0.956	0.912
IV	0.964	0.956	0.942	0.870
V	0.946	0.935	0.900	0.700
VI	0.875	0.845	0.680	0.000
VII	0.677	0.564	0.000	−1.486
VIII	−1.028	n.a.	n.a.	n.a.

Fixed points: Healthy = 1 Dead = 0

See Kind, Rosser and Williams 1982.
Source: Gudex 1986.

6 Clinical budgeting: experimentation in the social sciences. A drama in five Acts

Dramatis personae

Researchers One, Two and Three: Three sociologists of science who are researching into the practical application of health economics.
A tape-recorder: A small machine (perhaps a Sony TCM 9) which plays tapes of a health economist being interviewed by sociologists.
A video-recorder: A VHS machine with monitor which plays tapes of health economists teaching clinicians health economics at a special weekend course.
Kathleen: A health economist working within the NHS.
Don: A health economist working in a university applied-research unit.
Iden Wickings: The Director of the King's Fund CASPE research unit.

Throughout the play, the words of the fictional Researchers are made up for this text except in Act IV where they are drawn from an interview transcript. The speeches of all other characters are taken verbatim from transcripts and texts collected in the course of the research.

Act I: An idea is born in a London cafe

It is about one year into the research project on health economics. Two of the researchers are seated in a cafe in London discussing over a cup of tea how the project is going. They have just carried out an interview with a health economist who works at the nearby King's Fund Hospital Trust. There is a tape-recorder on the table. As the researchers talk they play back parts of the interview they have just recorded.

Researcher One: Well that seemed to go okay, it was friendly and relaxed and we got lots of anecdotes and good quotes we can use.

Researcher Two: Yes, he certainly was talkative. I think it definitely helped that you knew him. How did you get to meet him?

Researcher One: On the cricket field.

Researcher Two: You're kidding.

Researcher One: Not at all. When I was at High Tech University we had this departmental cricket team and every summer we would go on a cricket tour to play Knowex University's Economics Department. When I first met him he was playing for them. When I say 'playing', that is a bit of a joke actually; he was the worst cricketer I ever met, even worse than me. I always remember my first sight of him. He was a legendary character and he wore this ridiculous floppy sun hat. I was sitting on the boundary waiting to bat and someone skied a catch towards him and sure enough he dropped it. Well it turned out he was a great drinker and raconteur. We've kept in touch ever since, but we've never talked about his career in health economics until now. What I found to be intriguing about the interview is that while we were having all that fun on the cricket field, the poor bloke was going through an existential crisis concerning his faith in economics. I had no idea.

Researcher Two: Yes, that was interesting. Let's listen to that bit of the interview again, shall we? We've got plenty of time before we need to leave for our train.

Researcher One: Okay, I'll just rewind the tape. It was somewhere near the beginning as I recall. Let's try it here.

Tape-recorder: . . . we were inteviewed on October the first, and paid from October the first. Essentially York had got some money from the DHSS for two projects, but it had come through a bit late, later than expected, possibly they hadn't got their act together, I don't know. And they certainly weren't getting much in the way of applications, so the fact that I was around was appealing. And I couldn't resist risk aversion, three years' money – good money – flat on the campus, so I caved in and got married. Did teaching hospital costs for three years or so . . .

Researcher One (stopping tape): I think it was after this stuff about how he worked at York, but let's listen on here for a while.

Researcher Two: I can't believe how easy it was to get a job in those days – the only applicant for the job! The last job I tried for had 200 applicants.

Tape-recorder: . . . a typical York project. That's to say, thought up on the train getting down to DHSS. No, I'm being unkind of course. A relatively sketchy protocol though. Let's put it that way. Not the sort of detail I found later in my career at St Doubtings. . . . We produced a report, we analysed some numbers, but I felt looking back on it now, the thing was on tick-over most of the time – we played a lot of sport in York. There's a tape running, what am I doing?

Cricket? You didn't play much cricket in those days?

Cricket not much, a lot of table tennis, dominoes . . .

Researcher Two (stopping and advancing tape): Do you ever stop talking about cricket? Let's get on to where he leaves York for Knowex.

Tape-recorder: . . . the idea was that some of the work I was doing on teaching hospitals would become a D.Phil. And really what got my career going was an aspect of a formula that preceded the RAWP formula for dishing out money . . . I got interested in that for no obvious reason. It was a bit peripheral to our work on teaching hospitals and I cranked out a paper on that which then eventually got published in *Applied Economics*. . . . That was enough to get a job at the University of Knowex. Straightforward lecturer in economics in 1974. And I had four years' bashing away there, undergraduate tutorials but keeping up the health thing . . .

Researcher One (advancing tape): A proper lecturing job with only one publication, and no PhD. Incredible! In sociology, even in the 1970s you needed a PhD and two books for what few jobs there were.

Tape-recorder: I moved to St Doubtings in '78, really becoming increasingly fed up with economic theory. Not so much with health economics . . . I still went along with a lot of Alan Williams's line in those days. I still thought that in the practical fields one could do something with economics fairly well. But I was disillusioned with mathematics and economic theory, which is, it's essentially a game, whatever comes out is what you put in . . . I remember having a sort of crisis of confidence, worrying that I wasn't doing the best for my students . . . I got so frustrated by it. It seemed so pointless to me . . . I actually started reading a copy of the latest edition of *American Economic Review* and working through the articles. . . . You know that was a complete waste of time: what have we discovered?

Why didn't you get your disillusionment earlier?

I was extremely seduced by economics . . . I first went to York, there I was, it was well taught, Williams and, I don't know whether you get to sit in on their lectures and so on, but Williams and Culyer are very clear teachers. I think they're very persuasive and I really, I swallowed the whole story. You know, if only the world was like Alan Williams, if only everyone analysed their decisions in this way, wouldn't it be a better place? So I think there is a nice internal logic about economics which helps, like a crossword puzzle – the different pieces fit together – whereas something like accountancy has a set of rules, largely arbitrary ones . . .

Researcher Two (pausing tape): Poor old accountants, they get it in the neck every time from the economists. But this is good stuff. We can use this in the book, especially the bit about if only the world was like Alan Williams wants it to be.

Tape-recorder: I began to ask myself . . . I had tenure at Knowex . . . do I really want to spend the rest of my life pounding away at this stuff, when it's clearly not getting anybody anywhere. And I think that's when I really started to get fed up . . . I mean something I was using in lectures came out in a very prestigious journal as a comment. There is just some obvious side point that I'd been using in lectures, it never occurred to me to publish it because it was so obvious. . . . And that contributed to my disillusionment. . . . There was a famous article . . . it was about bargaining and where economics missed out on things, like concentrating on a simple fair trade model . . . [this] paper said that if you were going to trade once with somebody . . . you can trade good commodities or bad commodities . . . then on the whole you would give the guy the duff commodity, because on the whole you assume that's what he is going to give you and your gains are maximized if you give him the duff one. . . . A professor of economics at Sussex wrote a paper pointing out that if there was an expectation of continued trade between the parties, then on the whole they would be nicer to each other. That's to say, you don't want to turn a customer off with a dud the first time, so you give him a good one. Now my wife, who had just given up work, said, 'You know, since I've been going to that greengrocer around the corner regularly, I get much better stuff than when I used to pop in occasionally on my way back from school'. I thought now, if that is such an obvious bit of common sense that my wife who is no economist but a perfectly sensible citizen, if that's something that can be spotted in that sort of way, then why are we publishing that sort of thing in the *Quarterly Journal of Economics*?

Researcher One (stopping tape): Presumably to get a job as an economist! Anyway you've got to admire him for having the courage of his convictions, giving up a university position to work as a health economist in an applied context. But, surprise, surprise, when he got there he found that there wasn't much that he could do either, because it turned out that issues were settled more by local political interests than by economics. There was a good bit on this later on. (*Advancing tape.*) Listen to this. He's talking about a health economics study of mobile X-ray screening which showed that the costs far outweighed the benefits because of the low numbers of cancers and TB cases spotted.

Tape-recorder: I mean looking for six of anything per thousand screened just doesn't seem like a good piece of public money.

So it's that kind of decision that you feel health economists could help with?

I used to, I think certainly yes when I moved . . . I hoped that the sort of research that I was doing would help.

But it didn't?

Well it doesn't . . . it's only more recently that I've come to the conclusion that it doesn't help; partly because of its failure to take on board the different interest groups . . . and I'm annoyed with myself for not seeing it earlier. I mean how could I? I'm annoyed with my own naivety if you like. How could I have ever believed that you would walk right into a meeting of different interest groups and say, here are the costs of doing this, and here are the benefits, and here are the courses of action, and we've decided that benefits exceed costs by most in this one, so will you all please agree. I mean it seems to be mad looking back, that it's incredibly stupid of me to ever fall for that . . .

Are you saying that a perfect world, or a better world would involve being able to go round a table, and showing them the figures, and coming to an agreement on the basis of . . . ?

Not any more. I used to think that. Now, I think that there's no such thing as a better world. I mean they're just different worlds in which different people manage to secure more of a service that they're interested in. And I fully understand now why those people defended the mass miniature X-ray service. If they were reassured by it, then okay, fair enough, that's a legitimate reason for trying to hang on to the service . . .

Researcher Two: He seems to have become increasingly disillusioned with health economics. What's he doing now working at the King's Fund?

Researcher One: They offer courses to clinicians and health service managers. That's why Kathleen was there.

Researcher Two: I got a hell of a shock bumping into her in the lift. I just didn't expect to meet another of our respondents there.

Researcher One: You did very well to remember her name. I recognized her from an HESG meeting but didn't have a clue who she was. Rewind the tape a bit, there was a very funny story at the start about consultancy. Before you arrived he got a phone call from the World Bank in Washington. They wanted to fly him over for a two-day consultancy. (*Researcher Two rewinds tape.*)

Tape-recorder: . . . it is all piggy-backed onto Griffiths – management, consultancy, advice . . . someone pays for a group of managers to come in and talk about their problems . . . a sort of mixture of consultancy, therapy, customized teaching.

How much health economics enters into it?

Not much. I do some sessions particularly on economic type things, but they're more really health service finance. I do stuff on clinical budgeting, it is something that all the managers want to know about. . . . Well I don't get phone calls from the World Bank all the time – just an accident. One of the reasons I'm – I wouldn't say I was successful – one of the reasons I'm popular is because I almost never say no. . . . I've done a little bit of background work for London Weekend TV a couple of times for *cash* – cash in hand. They wanted some big numbers. What will AIDS cost in 1993 if we don't act now? Like a lot of economics you collect some numbers on cost, unit cost, and you collect some numbers on numbers of units and you sit there and multiply them and out comes your fee. . . . With London Weekend TV it was particularly nice because one of the guys providing the numbers kept changing his mind. So they were on the phone to him for ages chatting, and I was sitting there at the other end of the phone with this London Weekend guy sweating. And I was just sort of, he thought I was working out the numbers, I was working out my fee . . .

Researcher One (laughing): Wonderful, we could use that in the 'Quick and Dirty' chapter or the media chapter. But listening to the tape makes me feel depressed.

Researcher Two: Because you never get any consultancy?

Researcher One: That's true, but no, I was being serious for a moment. It's such a mess this health economics study. These people are just out there in the messy real world and it's a problem making sense of it all, trying to get a handle on things. I mean how do we treat this last interview? Was it with an 'insider' or an 'outsider'? Is he even a health economist at all as he seems to have given up serious research in health economics?

Researcher Two: Well most of the health economists we have talked with have claimed not to be proper health economists. That seems to be part of the character of health economics – it's either what you used to do or what someone else is doing.

Researcher One: But then how are we going to conclude anything? In a way, his current view – which is that political interests are more important than economics in understanding the NHS – is closer to our own view, but if he has ceased to be an economist, what weight can we give to his views? It wasn't like this when I studied physicists. You never got physicists saying, 'Well actually I'm not really a physicist' or 'I gave up physics because it was no better than common sense', or 'I now see that physics is all about social and political factors'. It was all so clear-cut. You found your experimentalist who claims to have observed a new phenomenon of the natural world and then you found a second who disagrees with the first and sees something completely different. And then you would interview both of them, along with their supporters and other protagonists. Finally, you showed there were good arguments on both sides and, hey presto! in comes the social world to settle matters. It was such a neat and tidy thing to do – all in the context of a tight technical argument over a small set of experiments, as Pinch (1986) did in his recent book. I really should have stayed with physics. Now we have these health economists who don't do experiments, and don't even claim to be health economists, and we waffle away for hours with them about the myriad problems of the NHS with a bit on their career, a bit on QALYs, a bit on option appraisal, a bit on measurement, a bit on rationality, and so on. You never know whether they really know what they're talking about or whether they're just talking off the tops of their heads. How on earth are we going to make sense of it all?

Researcher Two: I really do think you are romanticizing a little about the sociology of the natural sciences. Take another read of some of the recent stuff by Gilbert and Mulkay (1984), Ashmore (1988, 1989), Pinch and Pinch (1988) or Mulkay on his own (1984, 1985). But that aside, surely the health economists' world is no more and no less messy than ours as sociologists of science? Take the origins of this project. As I recall, we decided on health economics as a topic after you phoned a health economist friend at High Tech who told you about the HESG and HEART, and since you only had two days in which to write the proposal, you thought let's study this because at least we have a convenient sampling frame. Typical back-of-the-envelope type thing I seem to recall.

Researcher One: Well let's forget about that and be thankful the tape-recorder isn't on!

Researcher Two: You also keep saying that so and so isn't a proper sociologist of science and that you yourself have changed your views on the sociology of science as you have moved between different research locations. And look at all the changes in emphasis we have had during the course of this project. We don't do experiments and we seem to manage alright; so why is it any worse for the health economists?

Researcher One: I see reflexivity is rearing its ugly head again. Rather than go into all those issues which are dealt with in Woolgar's (1988) new collection, why don't you find me a nice clean-cut area of health economics, rather like scientific experiments, which I could feel comfortable about studying.

Researcher Two: How about clinical budgeting?

Researcher One: Oh, you mean the thing that all these managers want to learn about and which is taught at the King's Fund? It's some sort of financial decision-making system to enable clinicians and managers to manage more efficiently isn't it?

Researcher Two: That's right and many health economists we have talked to seem to be enthusiastic about it. But as usual the people involved sometimes deny being health economists.

Researcher One: But how is clinical budgeting like science? Surely budgeting is what you and I do when we come down to London and we have to decide whether we can afford British Rail sandwiches or a meal out on the research project.

Researcher Two: I think the health economists would say there was more to it than that. But on the train down I read this interesting article about experiments on clinical budgeting. It was in a health economics journal with an editorial by Tony Culyer.

Researcher One: Tony Culyer, he's one of the leading lights in health economics at York, right?

Researcher Two: Yes, that's the person. I have the journal in my briefcase. (*Researcher Two fumbles under the table for his briefcase and pulls out a battered copy of the journal* Nuffield/York Portfolios. *He opens it and starts to read out loud.*) 'Despite the three recent major organizational changes in the National Health Service the most striking features that continue to characterize its management are the absence of *variety in experimentation* in alternative ways of getting things done. . . . This folio reports on what is the one outstanding exception to these deficiencies: some real experiments in offering clinicians budgetary *incentives* to be better managers. Their importance is scarcely to be underestimated, given the uniqueness of such ordinary experiments in Britain. Iden Wickings and James Coles make the ethical case for clinical budgeting in the NHS and show how it links up with new developments in the provision of information for management at all levels' (Culyer 1985a: 1). Well this seems to be all about experimentation so why not have a look at it.

Researcher One: Pass it over. (*Researcher Two hands over the journal and Researcher One starts to read.*) It certainly does sound as if this is what I have been looking for. Wickings and Coles say that 'There have now been many clinical budgeting experiments in Britain' (Wickings and Coles 1985: 4). And this guy Wickings seems to have been involved with most of them. It says here that there were some very recent experiments carried out by Wickings which were highly influential in persuading the Griffiths Inquiry into health service management to advocate the introduction of management and clinical budgeting. They report that 'A more basic method of reaching . . . agreement [between clinicians and management] has recently been tested in some clinical budgeting experiments. The method involved district managers and clinicians negotiating *Planning Agreements with Clinical Teams* (PACTs)'. (*Researcher One giggles as he recognizes the awful pun.*) 'In early 1985 an independent Evaluation Group chaired by Professor Buller, the previous Chief Scientist at the DHSS concluded, "The evaluation group is not aware of any other system than PACTS that offers similar interaction between managers and clinicians" ' (ibid.: 7). Blah, blah. It seems that these experiments were a success. It goes on to say, 'The Evaluation Group is unanimously of the view that in principle this PACTs-centred budgeting system has all the right ingredients for improved resource management in the NHS, and it should be given the support needed to ensure its wider dissemination within the service' (ibid.: 7). This is great. I will have to get hold of that report on these successful experiments. Perhaps there are some critics somewhere we can track down. We might even have an experimental dispute as in physics.

Researcher Two: Are you happy now?

Researcher One: Well happiness is asking too much. But at last we are going to be able to deconstruct some real science instead of all these pseudo-scientific measures such as QALYs, option appraisals and the like which no one takes seriously. (*Looking at watch.*) Good grief! Look at the time. Come on. We'll have to shift if we want to catch the 5.30 train back to York.

Researcher Two: Aren't you forgetting one thing?

Researcher One: What's that?

Researcher Two: We said we would work out how much of the research budget we had left to spend before deciding whether we could afford a meal on the train.

Researcher One: That's right, but we've got no time to do it now. We're bound to have some money left in the kitty and there's no point in slumming it. I feel it's been such a productive day. I even think we might stretch to a bottle of wine on the train back. (*They hastily pay for their cup of tea and leave.*)

Act II: What is clinical budgeting?

Researcher Two is seated at his desk at the University of York staring at a video monitor. It is paused on a frame showing a health economist gesticulating at a large table of figures drawn on a blackboard. Researcher One enters carrying an envelope file of papers under his arm.

Researcher One: Morning. Mind if I disturb you for a bit?

Researcher Two: Not at all. I've been working on the 'Rationalized Choice' chapter, trying to read some of the figures from an option appraisal Don presented at that clinicians' course which I videoed. It's starting to give me a headache, and anything for a break.

Researcher One: It's on health economics again I'm afraid.

Researcher Two: The clinical budgeting chapter?

Researcher One: That's right. I got hold of that CASPE report, you know the one in which Wickings and his team present the results of their experiments. That document is dynamite. I can't really believe what I'm reading, so I just want to go through a few of the points with you to make sure I've got it right. I've started to write it all up for a talk I'm meant to be giving at Brunel University.

(*There is a knock at the door. Researcher Three enters.*)

Researcher Three: Mind if I join you? I need a break from administration.

Researcher One: Sure. We were just about to go through some of my material on clinical budgeting. I'm glad you've popped by because I'm drafting something to present to a seminar at Brunel University and this is an ideal opportunity to try it out on you both. There may be some health economists in the audience and I want to make sure I've understood the basic idea of clinical budgeting. Can I read you the start of the paper?

Researcher Three (sitting down): I'll imagine I'm an economist. Go ahead.

Researcher One (taking a typewritten manuscript from the file he reads out loud): 'Clinical budgeting and its close relation, management budgeting are financial decision-making systems which are intended to give users of health care resources, and in particular clinicians, a greater degree of choice over how resources are allocated such that, overall, resources may be used in a more efficient way' (Pinch, Ashmore and Mulkay 1987: 15).

Researcher Two: Sorry to interrupt you, but what justification is there for treating management and clinical budgeting as the same thing?

Researcher One: I'm glad you asked me that. As far as I can see they are essentially the same thing from the point of view of economics except that the emphasis in the two systems is slightly different. Overall they are both ways of planning a budget so as to make clinicians and managers more aware of costs and thus more efficient. In clinical budgeting the prime target is clinicians. There are powers of virement . . .

Researcher Two: Virement? What on earth's that?

Researcher One: It's the ability to transfer a surplus from one category to balance a deficit under another head. If a saving is made, the money can be spent on something else the clinicians think is desirable. Clinical budgeting has virement as a direct incentive to clinicians. Management budgeting, on the other hand, doesn't offer clinicians the same powers of virement. There are also differences in the ways the costing is done. In management budgeting costs include overhead costs such as rates or the cost of running the boiler house. The costing information is generally less accurate.

Researcher Two: They sound rather different to me and I'm not certain you are justified in lumping them together. Perhaps you should look at the ways in which for some purposes they are treated as the same and for other purposes as different.

Researcher One: Look, as usual you are trying to be too sophisticated. I want you to react as an economist might react. From the economist's point of view they are the same thing. I envisaged this might be a problem, so just to back me up, I found this article by Wickings in the *Health Service Journal* where he addresses precisely this issue. (*Researcher One takes another paper from his file.*) Let me quote you the man himself: 'Are management budgets different from clinical budgets? Clinical budgets have been under test in several countries for a number of years. In the NHS the CASPE Research Unit now has three experiments in progress. . . . The clinical budgets now in use have many features in common with management budgets although there are a few differences' (Wickings 1983: 466). He then goes on to say what exactly these differences are: 'To summarise, the differences are small although they possibly could be significant. None the less the approaches are sufficiently similar for most of us to ignore the finer distinctions' (ibid.: 467). I take that as a warrant to ignore the differences for the purposes of introducing clinical budgeting in my paper.

Researcher Two: Yes, but as we know, Wittgenstein said that all similarity and difference judgements are accomplished by us and similarities and differences don't reside out there.

Researcher One (exasperated): Of course, everything may seem either different or similar, but that is the kind of nuance which I just don't want to take up here.

Researcher Three: If I may interrupt. It seems to me that both of you are right.

Researchers One and Two: That's really helpful!

Researcher Three: Let me explain. It is clearly the case that any two things can be seen to be either similar or different. But whether you do 'similarity work' or 'difference work' depends on the practical occasion at hand. Presumably, for the practical purpose of presenting a paper to economists, you should treat management budgeting and clinical budgeting as the same thing. Similarly, for the practical task of his article, Wickings was warranted in treating the differences as being negligible. But it is also quite correct to point out, as he did, that for other purposes the differences could become quite crucial.

Researcher One: Well, given the preference to seek agreement in conversations, this is probably a good point for me to return to reading my paper. I only want you to judge whether health economists would find my account plausible, that's all.

Researcher Two: In other words, you want us to stop raising all the interesting issues. But as that is what economists also seem to want, you're probably on the right track.

Researcher One (reading): 'In the context of hospitals, where clinical budgeting is initially being introduced, rather than Health Authorities making a yearly allocation of resources to functional budgets – so much to pharmacy, so much to radiology, and so on – budgets will be allocated to each major area of clinical activity. This means that individual clinicians (and ward sisters) will have a greater part in deciding the resource allocation for the budgetary year. Clinicians need to be provided with information on how much different components of clinical activity cost (e.g. the costs of an X-ray, of a test done in a pathology laboratory, and so on) and on how much of their budget they have spent. This information is provided by new computer systems' (Pinch, Ashmore and Mulkay 1987: 15).

That all seems perfectly straightforward I hope. 'Clinical budgeting is held to be a way of achieving a more "rational" and "efficient" distribution of scarce resources such that ultimately patient care will be improved. Underlying the new decision-making systems is the view of social behaviour which is prevalent in economics, and it is no accident that the leading proponents of clinical budgeting within the UK have been health economists. According to economists, given scarce resources, individuals make choices in which they trade-off the costs of some action against benefits such as to maximize the benefits for themselves or for some group they purport to represent. The problem for health economists is that in this case the allocation of scarce resources cannot be mediated by the usual mechanism of market prices. This is because it is held that health care should not depend upon the ability to pay. Health economists are thus forced to search for surrogates for market prices. One way round the difficulty is to treat the consumption of resources by groups other than patients – such as clinicians – as the mediators of market forces. This is, in effect, the basis of the economic rationale for clinical budgeting' (ibid.: 16–18).

I then give a little quote from a health economist supporting this underlying economic rationale. I go on to say: 'The argument is that the system as a whole will operate most efficiently when benefit is being maximized by clinicians – clinicians in this case act, as it were, on behalf of their patients. As Wickings and Coles write, ". . . the clinicians can be given extra discretion and thus have an incentive to use their allocated resources more efficiently in the interests of their own clinical service and their patients. In this way optimizing the *output* of the NHS, in terms of quality and quantity of the service provided" (Wickings and Coles 1985: 3). In short, the rationale underlying clinical budgeting is none other than the standard route which economists offer for reaching Nirvana (that perfectly rational society in which the greatest good to the greatest number is produced by individuals trading-off costs and benefits and maximizing benefit)' (Pinch, Ashmore and Mulkay 1987: 18–19). That's it so far. Does that seem okay?

Researcher Two: I'm sure you're right that health economists do advocate clinical budgeting – our interviews support that. But I still have worries about you presenting a definitive version of clinical budgeting as if it was all based upon economic principle. I was looking the other day at the video of the talk on management budgeting which Kathleen gave at the course for clinicians. As I recall, she says hardly anything at all about economic principle. Instead, she put it all in terms of the practical problems which management budgeting helps to solve.

Researcher Three: Is that on the same tape you have just been looking at?

Researcher Two: Yes, it's after this option appraisal stuff. Shall we have a look? (*Advancing tape.*)

Researcher One: I really want to get onto the testing of clinical budgeting as soon as possible. That's the bit that interests me because it's most like physics.

Researcher Two: This is the sort of thing I mean. Here is Don, who chaired the session, introducing Kathleen:[1]

Video-recorder: . . . it's also relevant, of course, because it's actually being imposed to a considerable extent on the service. And so exactly what is the sort of experience that have, there have been so far? They are both highly relevant questions and they'll be questions to which Kathleen will be addressing herself this morning.

Researcher Two (stopping and advancing tape): See what I mean? He seems to be emphasizing the practical side of knowing about something that is going to come into force anyway. Kathleen's introduction is also in terms of her practical experience with management budgeting. Listen to this:

Video-recorder: Every district has to commence implementation . . . and we went out to district and worked with districts and helped them implement management budgeting. . . . So if your district is starting on the path of implementing management budgeting, these are the sorts of area you might find yourself being involved in.

Researcher Two (stopping and advancing tape): Then she uses all the rhetorical devices we are familiar with from our 'Colonizing the Mind' chapter. She disassociates management budgeting from cost cutting, and, of course, it's nothing to do with accountancy.

Video-recorder: . . . this is *very very* important. Management budgeting is *not* a costing system, it's not a glorified cost accountancy system, it's about *management*, managing resources . . .

Researcher Three: That's a lovely example of a three-part list with a contrast. In other words, two things which management budgeting *isn't* are presented, followed by a third thing which it *is*. And look how each point is accompanied by a downward arm movement to add emphasis. She is using all the skills of political rhetoric which Max Atkinson (1984) documents.

Researcher Two (advancing tape): Later on she claims management budgeting is all about helping patients:

Video-recorder: Also it's quite specifically patient related, in other words you're looking at the sort of things you can deliver to patients, it makes sense to the consultants, to the doctors, it also makes sense to the nurses, because under management budgeting we actually have a system of ward budgets and consultant budgets.

Researcher One: It seems as though it is designed to help just about everyone.

Researcher Two (advancing tape): And the implications are only to be felt at the margins.

Video-recorder: And a lot of – in my experience – a lot of consultants actually, are happy with what they're doing now and they just want, you know, want to make sure they're not going to get squeezed. But you know they just chug along and maybe in a few years time they'll make some more changes . . . I mean I'm sure that Don is saying what you know, that most of the changes are at the margins. A great body of your costs are fixed, it is quite difficult to change . . .

Researcher Three: It seems to be rather like the distinction between the strong and weak programmes of health economics which we outlined in the 'Colonizing the Mind' chapter. Kathleen and Don when they talk to clinicians present management budgeting as something which will help them do what they do already a little better. It involves no radical change and effects things only at the margin. It is very much in the vein of the weak programme.

Researcher One: It's what we might call a 'user friendly' system.

Researcher Two: That's a good metaphor. After all, one of the main features of clinical budgeting is its use of computers which doctors fear will feed yet more useless information into the NHS. Kathleen addresses this point specifically (*rewinding tape*).

Video-recorder: . . . it sounds horrible. I've just been on a planning course at the King's Fund last week, and we've sort of had all this wonderful management jargon thrown at us, you know, and you can open your mouth and out it comes . . .

Researcher Two (stopping tape): Sorry that's the wrong place.

Researcher One: That must have been the course at the King's Fund which she was attending when we met her a few weeks ago. I'm really starting to feel part of this network.

Researcher Two (rewinding tape some more): I think this is the right place now.

Video-recorder: . . . the point is, you must have a budget statement that is accessible to you, that is interesting to you, that gives *you* the sort of information that you want.

Researcher Three: Does she ever stop using three-part lists?

Researcher Two (advancing tape): Her talk is full of them. Here is another where she argues that what consultants want is more flexibility – a flexibility which of course management budgeting provides them with.

Video-recorder: . . . and as consultants we want the ability to get our hands *more* on the budget, we want *more* flexibility, we want to be able to actually change more within what we're doing . . .

Researcher Two: This version of management budgeting seems to be a long way away from the attempt at radical change in clinicians' behaviour which you propose at the start of your Brunel paper. (*Advancing tape.*) Here is just one last statement from her as to what it is. This is probably the weakest version of all.

Video-recorder: Management budgeting isn't a panacea; management budgeting isn't going to solve your problems. What it is, it's a searchlight on the management problems . . .

Researcher Three: I don't believe it, another three-part list and contrast formulation.

Researcher One: Yes, I'm sure he's selecting the data so that we only listen to lists and contrasts.

Researcher Two: Not at all, but I must admit when I went through the tape the other day I marked the places on the counter which I thought might interest us.

Researcher Three: If I may summarize. There is a radical economic rationale or 'strong programme' of clinical budgeting which we have used at the start of the Brunel paper, and then there is a 'weak programme' of trying to help clinicians with their problems and attending to their misconceptions about these kinds of budgeting systems. And it is this latter version which is presented by Kathleen in her talk.

Researcher Two: Maybe she takes a rather different line in her presentation at that recent HESG session on clinical budgeting.

Researcher One: I really feel we should move on to the CASPE study, we seem to be getting side-tracked.

Researcher Two: No, this is important because if Kathleen presents management budgeting in a different way there we can start to document how management budgeting is a flexible resource which actors present in different ways for the particular occasion at hand.

Researcher One: Well, her talk at the HESG is not a very easy thing to analyse because as you may remember she spends most of her time countering another health economist, Peter West, who raised eighteen different objections to clinical budgeting.

Researcher Two: Do you by any chance have a copy of the relevant documents with you?

Researcher One (searching in the folder): This is Peter's paper called 'Clinical budgeting: A critique'. And Vivienne has just finished the transcript of Kathleen's response and the subsequent discussion. There may be a few words she didn't get but as usual it's good enough to work from.

Researcher Two: How does Peter present clinical budgeting?

Researcher One: Well rather in the same way that I presented it in my paper for Brunel. In fact it was Peter who was the health economist I quoted in the introduction to my paper. He said: 'The central plank of clinical budgeting is that if the use of services was charged to a clinician's budget, higher cost services would be reflected in a faster depletion of the budget, forcing consultants and other doctors to choose between a reduced level of activity and a reduced use of resources for each case. This is precisely the model that economists use in examining consumer behaviour in the market place' (West 1986: 2).

Researcher Two: But he's *criticizing* clinical budgeting there, so how do you know that his version is the definitive one?

Researcher One: Well, as I said before, he simply puts forward the economic view underlying the whole thing, so I would have thought that it was largely uncontentious.

Researcher Two: But the whole point is that you can talk about it in a way that Kathleen did without ever having to mention this economic rationale.

Researcher Three: Perhaps we can settle this by seeing how Kathleen responded to Peter's criticisms.

Researcher One: Okay, but as I seem to remember her response was pretty weak. She doesn't seem to take on board any of his economic arguments. But we're wasting time. The important thing is to move on to the testing of clinical budgeting. We don't want to get bogged down in these nuances of presentation. (*Researcher One passes transcript over and says testily:*) But if you are so keen, you have a look at it.

Researcher Two (reading through transcript): Well, here's something interesting for a kick off. She says: 'I mean we're starting to get into problems already because he seems to use clinical budgeting and management budgeting interchangeably. I've gone back to Griffiths and I think that we're quite clear about what we're talking about'.[2]

Then she quotes Peter as saying that 'the main objective of clinical budgeting is to increase efficiency'. But according to her, 'That is not the case. I mean if you go back again to your Griffiths then management budgeting is very much about management and it's about accountability. Increasing efficiency is not in my view the main view of clinical budgeting'. In other words, there is a genuine dispute over the *meaning* of clinical budgeting or management budgeting, call it what you will, at a very fundamental level. In summarizing her comments on Peter she says, '. . . what he's saying essentially is nothing really much to do with management budgeting . . . he's missing the point about management budgeting in Griffiths, which is about management and accountability'. By the same token you missed the point about clinical budgeting in the introduction to your paper for Brunel.

Researcher One: I can't take Kathleen seriously. I mean, who is this 'Griffiths' she keeps harking back to? Is he the Isaac Newton of health economics or perhaps the Albert Einstein? No, he's Roy Griffiths, a manager of a big supermarket chain! And no one at the HESG took her seriously either. Look at the transcript; Peter puts her down to devastating effect (*reading transcript*): 'Now, Kathleen says it wasn't intended to increase efficiency, but it was intended to increase accountability and responsibility. It seems to me that, I mean what is it, why are you trying to increase accountability if not to increase efficiency? Why are you trying to make people more responsible? You've overspent £5,000 – congratulations (*laughter*)'.

Researcher Three: Notice the use of the three-part joke format, building up a puzzle in a list of three. It's no wonder he got masses of laughter.

Researcher Two: It seems to me that you're taking Peter's side against Kathleen and you simply can't do that because the 'correct' view is what is precisely at stake. They are both reputable health economists who are very familiar with clinical budgeting and to take one side would be to prejudge the issue.

Researcher Three: Perhaps we can go back to this weak programme/strong programme idea. Did Kathleen's version of clinical budgeting presented to the HESG differ from that which she presented to the clinicians?

Researcher One: As I've said, it's quite hard to tell because at the HESG she was very much on the defensive in response to Peter's attack. However, I did notice one startling change. If you recall when talking to the clinicians, she stressed that management budgeting was designed only to bring about changes at the margin. But she said exactly the opposite at the HESG. Listen to this: 'I think another problem with management budgeting is just seeing it as being movements at the margin. . . . And *again* I think that misses the point as to what we're trying to do, and what Griffiths is trying to do; he's trying to look at the totality of resource allocation and management of those resources. And I think that concentrating at the margin just isn't really what the core of the issue is. I feel it's a very narrow view'.

Researcher Three: That's interesting. Kathleen certainly seems to go for a stronger version of management budgeting when arguing with Peter West at the HESG.

Researcher Two: Which is exactly my point. If there is no one definitive version of clinical budgeting, how can we present one at Brunel?

Researcher One: Listen, we have been through all this before. At Brunel I'll be talking to health economists not clinicians, so the 'strong programme' version is the one that is appropriate.

Researcher Two: I just find it odd that we as sociologists can feel happy about changing our versions of what clinical budgeting is about to suit different audiences.

Researcher Three: But if the economists manage to do it, why shouldn't we as sociologists also do it? But I think we're all getting tired and could do with a coffee. I feel it's been a very productive session.

Researcher One: Well that's debatable. Perhaps I can tell you about the CASPE tests of clinical budgeting over coffee. (*Researchers all get up and leave office for coffee bar.*)

Act III: The problems of experimentation

The three researchers are seated around a table drinking coffee. Researcher One has a document spread out on the table in front of him to which he refers as he talks.

Researcher One: The results are contained in this report entitled *Experiments Using PACTs in Southend and Oldham HAs*. HAs are, of course, Health Authorities. It's written by Iden Wickings, Timothy Childs, James Coles and Claire Wheatcroft and is produced by the CASPE research unit of King Edward's Hospital Fund – better known as the King's Fund.

Researcher Three: I know what the King's Fund is but what does CASPE stand for?

Researcher One: These health economists love their acronyms. CASPE stands for Clinical Accountability, Service Planning and Evaluation. It is a sub-unit of the King's Fund. It seems to have been established by the DHSS as a separate unit to carry out targeted research such as that on clinical budgeting.

Researcher Three: And just to fill me in, when was the report produced?

Researcher One: It came out in December 1985. That is seven years after the research was funded by the DHSS in 1978. The project actually started in 1979.

Researcher Three: Was it a large amount of funding?

Researcher One: Well it was enough for Wickings to head a research team consisting of three staff with nine additional research team leaders located in the field at three different NHS Districts. That, on anyone's reckoning, is a sizable operation. The funding was, for instance, about ten times larger than the grant we've got for our research on health economics. Incidentally, I see that Kathleen is listed here as one of the research team leaders.

Researcher Two: She seems to turn up everywhere.

Researcher Three: Are these experiments the first of their kind in the UK?

Researcher One: Yes, but a clinical budgeting system has been in operation at Johns Hopkins University Hospital in the States for the past fifteen years, and several European countries are also experimenting with clinical budgeting. However, given the peculiarities of health care systems in different countries, such experiments haven't played much part in the UK debate.

Researcher Three: I see. Is this Wickings's first shot at this type of experiment?

Researcher One: Wickings took part in two earlier small-scale studies in this country. The first was at Westminster Hospital and was the prototype for his current work. Clinicians managed their own budgets and this led to some savings being made. In his second study in Brent health district, rather than give the clinicians budgets, he only provided them with information on costs, and this proved to be less successful. Although, as we shall shortly see, what success means in this game is far from obvious.

Researcher Three: And just to make sure I've got it absolutely clear, it is this study reported on here which led to the Griffiths Inquiry advocating what they called management budgeting?

Researcher One: Absolutely. The Griffiths Inquiry team visited Wickings's experiments whilst they were still in progress and they were so impressed by what they saw that they recommended the implementation of management budgeting in their report. Now twenty so-called 'demonstration districts' have been set up to further the implementation programme. Wickings has also continued to do his own follow-up studies, and in particular one at Guy's Hospital.

Researcher Three: Given what we said earlier about the strong and weak programmes of health economics, how is Wickings's report couched? Is clinical budgeting presented merely as something to help clinicians overcome their practical difficulties or is a rather stronger brew offered?

Researcher One: Well let me answer that by telling you my own reactions to reading the report. As you know when I first got hold of it I was excited because it looked like real science. As its title indicates, it seemed to be all about experiments. The original proposal made to the DHSS was formulated to answer specific questions, the central three being (*reading*): '(i) Can the Westminster/Brent budgetary system for consultants be established in very different districts? (ii) If so, what happens? (iii) What general conclusions can be drawn?' (Wickings *et al.* 1985: 4). It was claimed that (i) and (ii) could be resolved by, it says here, 'direct observation' (ibid.: 5). The report as a whole is heavy with this sort of scientific rhetoric. Technical terms are defined carefully, it is written up in the format of a scientific report with sections on 'The Experiments in Outline' and 'Results from the First Phase Experiments' and, as you can see here, it is full of graphs, tables and figures. There was, however, one oddity which I noticed. This is an early section of the report entitled 'Evaluation'.

Researcher Three: Research evaluation is quite a standard thing in applied social science projects, particularly in the States.

Researcher One: That may be so, but I was puzzled about why *experiments* needed external evaluation. Usually, the experimenter's interpretation of results is all that is required.

Researcher Three: Does it give any special reason why additional evaluation was felt to be desirable?

Researcher One: Well, part of the evaluation process involved getting the views of the participants in the experiments, but the more interesting aspect was the setting up of a special Evaluation Group to monitor developments. It says here that 'It was also proposed that the DHSS should itself establish an evaluation group, from which it will receive advice and a report' (ibid.: 5).

Researcher Two: Is that the same group headed by the Government Chief Scientist which reported so favourably on the experiments and which was cited in that Wickings and Coles (1985) article in the *Nuffield/York Portfolio* – the article which got you started on this whole thing?

Researcher One: Yes, that's it. The group consisted of a number of senior health service managers, a professor of health economics, a professor of accountancy, a senior medic, a regional nursing officer and a regional medical officer.

Researcher Two: In short, all the interest groups likely to be concerned with the introduction of clinical budgeting.

Researcher Three: Apart from patients.

Researcher One: Yes quite, but of course every interest group claims to speak for patients! Anyway, getting back to the Evaluation Group, at their first meeting held in October 1980, they decided that there might be a conflict of interest between steering and evaluating the project. It was therefore agreed that their remit should be evaluation only. It says, 'The Group's major role is to evaluate the outcome of the CASPE project – that is to say make a judgement as to whether the value of the clinical service planning and budgeting approach justifies the cost likely to be involved in setting up the budgetary arrangements. It is hoped that when the project is completed the Group will be in a position to recommend to the Department whether the approach should be commended for more general use in the service' (ibid.: 6). That last point is highly significant because, of course, it is exactly that sort of recommendation which the Griffiths Inquiry team made. But the Evaluation Group had another role to play: 'The Department recommended that if, in the final analysis, the Evaluation Group considered the clinical budgeting research to be of value, it would be essential to widely advertise the results, thereby allowing other districts to adopt a similar management style. The Evaluation Group would therefore have an important role to play in the dissemination of the research results . . .' (ibid.: 7). Not only were they evaluating the research, and making recommendations for future policy, but they were also responsible for publicizing the findings. Provided, of course, the findings were positive. I never encountered anything quite like this with the physicists I studied. It is as if, in a particular area of science, the scientists, their funders and the science media were all rolled up into one with the power to determine the future development of that area.

Researcher Two: It could be the case that in applied areas of science this is the way things work. If you think of tests of new technologies such as a new aeroplane, it is so complex and there are so many interests at stake that there is bound to be some official evaluation process.

Researcher One: Yes, that may be so. But what I don't see is why the decision over whether or not the thing works has to be connected to its exploitation. First, you want to know if you have a genuine effect; then, if there seem to be practical applications, you can seek funds from industry or support from the government, and, if you feel you need it, you can always work up some publicity. The priority, however, must be on the researchers' right and ability to decide first whether the experiments work as claimed.

Researcher Two: Distance really does lend enchantment, doesn't it? The less involved you get with research on physics, the more your depiction of how things work there relies on what you used to dismiss as old-fashioned views of the natural sciences. Work in the sociology of science, such as Latour's (1987) for example, has challenged every one of these points. It just isn't the case that ideas are developed in a 'pure' context which are then taken up later for purposes of 'application'.

Political interests and media interests are often there right from the start, even in physics. Look at the current fuss over the search for room-temperature superconductors, for instance.

Researcher One: I suppose I've got to say reluctantly that you're right. But you must agree that Robert Millikan never needed an 'Evaluation Group' to sit over him to decide whether his measurements of the charge of the electron were worth pursuing.

Researcher Two: And probably just as well too! Gerald Holton's (1978) research on Millikan's notebooks shows how Millikan rejected lots of measurements with deviant values that didn't fit his preconceptions of what the charge should be. If he had had an Evaluation Group watching his every move they might have noticed that what was to become one of the most celebrated experiments in physics was actually inconclusive! But joking aside, you shouldn't be comparing clinical budgeting experiments with basic science experiments. A better comparison is with technologies which are being tested in a public context. I don't know much about it, but from my reading of historians of technology such as Edward Constant (1980), it seems to be the case that new technologies are often tested in a very public forum – especially when the public might need to be persuaded to take up the technology. The trials of the first turbine driven boat, the *Turbina*, were held in public. And if you are really interested in pursuing the analogy, Harry Collins (1988) has recently sent me a preprint on a couple of cases involving public testing: one was of the transportation of a nuclear waste flask by train; the CEGB staged a public crash to show how safe it was. The other case Harry looked at was the testing of an additive to kerosene to stop aircraft fires being so devastating. Again, a mock crash was staged. Both are cases of tests where there were technical experts and the media present to evaluate the results.

Researcher One: Are you saying that these clinical budgeting experiments are more like the testing of a technology than scientific experimentation?

Researcher Two: Well, in a way. You can argue, for example, that health economics is a social technology. Clinical budgeting involves an attempt to change human behaviour using the principles of economics and, as a system, includes material artefacts such as computers and software packages. Indeed, there is a lot of new work in the sociology of technology which argues that all technologies are irretrievably a mixture of social, material, economic and political elements – a 'seamless web' is how it is described in the book by Bijker, Hughes and Pinch (1987).

Researcher One: I like the idea of health economics as a technology. It means that we can present this material to the sociology of technology people and get an additional audience for our research. But going back to the Evaluation Group for a moment, it does seem to be different from those very public tests you mentioned. For one thing it was all kept under wraps by the DHSS, who appointed the Group in the first place, and it was, of course, run by their own chief scientist. The Evaluation Group in this case seems to have acted as a buffer between the experiment and the wider public and policy contexts. If you recall it was the recommendation of the Evaluation Group which was cited by Wickings and Coles (1985: 7) in their article rather than the results reported here (*pointing to report on table*).

Researcher Two: The Evaluation Group can thus be seen as a neat way of giving an authoritative public interpretation of the experiments without having to address the messy and potentially defeasible process of the research itself. And, of course, the fact that the Group is formally independent from the experimenters gives it even more authority – which is why Wickings and Coles cite the report of the Evaluation Group rather than their own findings. As I'm sure you are both aware, this is yet another instance of the well-established finding of the sociology of science that distance lends enchantment to scientific certainty. The further you are away from the messy details of laboratory work, the more certain the results appear to be. The Evaluation Group in this case was able to transform the messy reality of experimental activity into a firm policy edict.

Researcher Three: Clearly we will have to study this Group further. But first I for one want to learn more about the experiments themselves; were they really that messy?

Researcher One: It was more than just a mess, it was a disaster. The most interesting thing about the report is that as I read it I became increasingly puzzled as to how the research could ever be seen as a success.

Researcher Three: It ran into difficulties then?

Researcher One: You can say that again. But before getting on to what those difficulties consisted of, let me tell you a little bit about how they planned to test the clinical-budgeting system.

Researcher Three (looking at report): I can see that it's full of these cursed acronyms. What on earth are CATs and DMTs?

Researcher One: CATs, or Clinically Accountable Teams, are the new formations in which clinicians are supposed to work. CATs have planned budgets which have previously been negotiated with the DMTs, the District Management Teams. The planning agreements with the DMTs are known as PACTs, which are Planning Agreements with Clinical Teams. All pretty straightforward isn't it? PACTs are the main feature of this type of clinical budgeting. A PACT is established each year which would set the budget for that year and outline the various clinical developments that were planned. As part of the project, CATs would be provided with extensive information as to what their various costs were. It says here that the CATs 'were to be afforded major opportunities to redeploy resources within their budgetary limits' (ibid.: 17). This is the basic economic rationale designed to change clinicians' behaviour which I outlined earlier. If the clinician has the responsibility for the budget he or she will spend the money in a more economically efficient way. There is much debate amongst health economists over the most effective form of incentive for clinicians, and in this form of clinical budgeting virement is the main incentive.

Researcher Two: This is the 'strong programme' of clinical budgeting?

Researcher One: Exactly. They then selected three particular districts of the NHS – Oldham, Southend and East Birmingham – in which to run the experiments. Similar districts were selected as controls.

Researcher Three: That seems fairly clear. So what does the report say?

Researcher One: Well, after setting out the aims of the research the report profiles the three different districts and outlines how the research was implemented in each of them. Great attention is given to what is called the 'Organizational Environment'. The reason for this is spelt out later where it says, 'During the five year period of the research a large number of fundamental changes occurred in the orientation of the NHS. In combination with the more usual factors such as staff changes and selective industrial action they provided an environment within which the research took place and against which the results should be evaluated' (ibid.: 18).

Researcher Three: It sounds as if they are hinting at problems to come.

Researcher One: That's right. And the first problem is a pretty damning one. Look, this is the chapter in which the results are given. They are prefaced by the statement that there will be no results from East Birmingham at all! This was apparently because the project had to be abandoned in that district before any discussions with clinicians were held.

Researcher Two: That looks to me like a pretty straightforward failure.

Researcher One: But the question is what counts as success or failure? Since the project at Birmingham never got started it could be treated as not properly a part of the experiment at all and therefore neither a failure nor a success.

Researcher Two: That sounds like gross ad hocery to me.

Researcher Three: Surely some sort of reason is advanced as to why that part of the experiment was abandoned?

Researcher One: It says here, 'There is almost no reference to the project in East Birmingham because (a) a separate report for the Evaluation Group has already been prepared and (b) the experiment was abandoned. . . . The abandonment was a decision taken by CASPE Research because the unit Director judged that the East Birmingham DMT was insufficiently committed to implementation within a reasonable time-scale. It should be noted, however, that the second of the recent NHS reorganisations was in progress at the time and this placed great difficulties upon the Districts concerned' (ibid.: 52).

Researcher Two: That sounds to me like a classic way of handling a negative result. It is a point which sociological studies of the natural sciences have repeatedly revealed. Since every experiment involves a whole host of background assumptions – *ceteris paribus* type clauses – the significance of any experimental result is in principle questionable. It can always be argued that some factor from the environment or some background theory was responsible for the negative result.

Researcher One: Right, that's the classic Duhem–Quine thesis: It's like what we used to do in our studies of physics when we showed how scientists actively negotiate what counts as background and what counts as foreground during the course of an experimental controversy. An experimenter claiming some new phenomenon of the natural world may face hostile critics who argue that some uncontrolled background effect is really responsible for the results. A good experimenter tries to rule out such potential grounds for criticism by producing as 'closed' an experiment as possible. A successful critic is one who manages to open up the experiment to the environment.

Researcher Two: But in this clinical budgeting case it is the experimenters themselves who are citing environmental factors – such as the NHS reorganization – to explain why a negative result is not actually a disconfirmation of the phenomenon.

Researcher Three: Aren't you two building a lot on what is after all only one small aspect of the report?

Researcher One: Oh, but it goes beyond just the Birmingham case. The results chapter as a whole is full of similar moves to accommodate negative results. For instance, the authors continually draw attention to the adverse environment they faced during the course of the experiment. It refers here to the 'worst of all environments in which to test' (ibid.: 53) and it goes on to list a number of organizational changes which took place at the time. But what I found to be so amazing about the report – and this is the real gen – was the section on the quantitative data. That is the real test of all this economic theorizing. If clinical budgeting was to have any effect then it should show up by changes in the resources used by clinicians. But as I read through the lists of all the quantitative measures examined I found that there was not a single number which could be said to show unambiguously that clinical budgeting was having an effect. The best that could be said was that the data were inconclusive.

Researcher Two: That *is* pretty amazing given that the whole point of clinical budgeting is to bring about changes in how clinicians use resources.

Researcher Three: I would like to know a little bit more about these quantitative measures.

Researcher One: Okay. The first thing they looked at were changes in non-staff clinically related items such as drugs, X-ray consumables and the purchase of medical equipment. They compared the costs in the experimental districts with the region as a whole. They found it a difficult exercise to do and were apparently unable to come to any clear conclusions (*reading*): '. . . perhaps the only firm conclusion that can be drawn is that it is impossible to make any such conclusions from this type of data' (ibid.: 86). They then looked for changes in resource use brought about by the specific PACT agreements. There are pages and pages of figures but again their conclusion was, 'In summary the figures do not conclusively demonstrate either a better or worse use of resources' (ibid.: 91). No firm conclusions could be drawn from data on patient management related costs or on case mixes either.

Researcher Two: I don't believe this. There must have been some positive results to report. Surely the Griffiths team can't have got it totally wrong.

Researcher One: Well, there is one positive result. Let me read you this: 'Although the analysis earlier in this chapter suggests that little happened which apparently changed the overall performance of the districts, when measured in terms of overall throughput or relative expenditure on particular headings, it is fair to point out that the PACT discussions between clinicians and members of the District Management Team were found to be worthwhile on a number of counts and that during these meetings a number of important planning issues were raised' (ibid.: 110). Basically they got on better! (*Laughter.*)

Researcher Two: That's really ironic. Their one success is in an area which seems to have little to do with economics. But this is all very puzzling; how on earth could these experiments be regarded in any way as a success?

Researcher One: That was exactly what I was trying to understand by the time I got to the section on 'Lessons Learnt'. Indeed, it seems that the authors of the report themselves realized that they faced something of a problem. They wrote at the start of this section, 'It sounds perverse, and may indeed be so, to regard the experiments reported here as encouraging rather than disappointing' (ibid.: 133). There follows a list of the 'encouraging' points. I must admit I chuckled reading this list. It goes as follows: '(i) The management teams in both Oldham and Southend have continued to invest in staff to support the system. (ii) Much technological development occurred which has since been adopted by the Management Budgeting demonstration districts'. Those, by the way, are the ones set up after the Griffiths Report. '(iii) Some (although the minority) of consultants liked and used the available systems and a number of beneficial changes were made'. These are the changes such as the 'talking together' which I referred to earlier. (*Laughter from Researchers Two and Three.*) '(iv) The ward sisters in Southend enjoyed being budget holders.' (*More laughter from Researcher Two.*) I thought you'd like that one. Here is another important finding: '(v) Mr Jim Blyth, of the Griffiths Inquiry team, was sufficiently impressed to advocate what he called "Management Budgeting" after his visit to Southend and the systems have substantial similarities.' You see they are alike after all! Now comes the finding to which they attach the most importance: '(vi) Perhaps of more significance, the national Evaluation Group were supportive in their interim report (April 1985).' If you recall, that is the positive report which Wickings and Coles quote in their article. Finally they say: '(vii) Although there were only limited signs of "success" there have been even fewer suggestions that the overall thrust was wrong' (Wickings and Coles 1985: 133–4).

Researcher Two (disbelieving): Is that it?

Researcher One: Yes that's it. After five years of experimentation that is what they found.

Researcher Two: Well, one thing I've learnt from this project is that in comparison the parapsychology experiments looked at by Collins and Pinch (1982) seem like Nobel Prize candidates!

Researcher One: I told you it was dynamite. The most interesting thing about this list, apart from its meagre nature in contrast with the original objectives, is that most of the positive reasons given are on the lines of saying it is a success because other people like it, or even, in the case of the Evaluation Group, because other people think that it's a success! That really does seem to put the cart before the horse. If there is no evidence that the thing works in the first place, you could argue that the more people that come to believe in it, the bigger is the failure.

Researcher Three: What was the exact statement which the Evaluation Group made in support?

Researcher One: Well, there is a lot of hedging around describing the experiments and so forth, but the key part is the last paragraph where it says, 'Despite the major difficulties encountered in the research districts, the Evaluation Group is unanimously of the view that in principle this PACTs-centred budgeting system has all the right ingredients for improved resource management in the NHS, and it should be given the support needed to ensure its wider dissemination within the service' (quoted in Wickings *et al.* 1985: 7).

Researcher Two: That sounds very positive to me. The 'in principle' caveat is a nice way of putting it. Of course, *in principle*, the system is the right one even if it doesn't work in practice. It is the classic way to save the phenomenon. If your experiment has been refuted you say that it wasn't actually a proper test and therefore the negative evidence doesn't count for anything. This puts a nice slant on an argument I recently read in a paper by Donald MacKenzie (1988) on the testing of ballistic-missile technology. MacKenzie points out that tests of strategic ballistic missiles off the coast of the United States can be challenged by saying that the results obtained there may not be applicable when the weapons are used in a real nuclear war. This argument was, for instance, made for a time by the US manned-bomber lobby. You challenge the positive results by pointing to a difference between the context of testing and the context of use. For those who wish to generalize from the tests, the context of test and context of use are held to be similar. But for the critics the differences are significant.

Researcher One: Back to similarity and difference judgements again?

Researcher Two: Exactly. The connection between testing and use can be said to be a matter of social negotiation. Our own case exhibits the same phenomenon but in a different way. Here we have a negative rather than a positive test result being discounted because it is claimed that the context of testing was in some way special because of major reorganizations of the NHS which took place during the test. In this case too it is claimed that the context of the test does not match the context of use. The Evaluation Group argue that under normal conditions of use there is every reason to believe that clinical budgeting will work properly. In short, the similarity and difference between context of use and context of test is again seen to be a flexible resource for argument.

Researcher Three: I think that what the two of you are saying is interesting but I am worried about one thing. In order to make this kind of argument at all, you have had to set up a definitive version of clinical budgeting – the version which says that it is an attempt to change economic behaviour and that whether or not it succeeds in doing so can be discovered by 'direct observation' in these experiments. You then deconstruct the Evaluation Group's 'success' claim by contrasting it with a 'failure' version which you derive from this report. But isn't there another way of looking at it? Suppose there is more than one version of clinical budgeting available. I seem to remember that one of you not so long ago was arguing this very case. Suppose we take the version of clinical budgeting which Kathleen presented to the clinicians which suggests that it is a modest attempt to offer practical help and that success is to be defined in terms of getting the thing working to however limited an extent. You wouldn't, of course, expect such marginal benefits to show up in the quantitative data. In terms of this version, rather than being a failure you can start to see how the experiments might be seen as a success, especially given the hostile environment at the time. The fact that people such as ward sisters liked the system – which you sneered at in that rather sexist way earlier – is actually as good a measure of success as anything else. The fact that it is taken up by practitioners is surely in the end the best criterion of success.

Researcher One: I see what you are saying, but my point is that it was the participants themselves, that is Wickings and co., who made the appeal to scientific rhetoric. And they themselves acknowledged that the experiments were less than successful; remember Wickings said, quote, 'It sounds perverse . . . to regard the experiments reported here as encouraging rather than disappointing'.

Researcher Three: Well, we will clearly have to talk to Wickings himself to get his view. It could be the case that these different rhetorics are continually drawn upon for different purposes. Even arguing that clinical budgeting is a technology seems to involve one particular version.

Researcher Two: I'm glad the stuff on technology was useful even if it did only highlight how we as analysts are using different versions of health economics. But I've got to get back to my video analysis. It's time for some real research.

Researcher One: You're forgetting. We've got to arrange some more interviews. We need to talk with Wickings and also somebody who was a member of this Evaluation Group.

Researcher Three (getting up to go): Well, I'll leave you both to do that. And if you find time, perhaps you could read through these two chapters which I've just finished. (*Handing over typescript.*) I've got to get back to some administration – another of these damn surveys evaluating the department has arrived.

Act IV: Wickings' world

The location is a large office resplendent with Edwardian furniture at the King's Fund Trust in London. Iden Wickings is seated behind a large desk. Researchers One and Two are seated in easy chairs in front of the desk. On the desk is a small tape-recorder.[3]

Researcher One: I wonder if you could just say a little bit about the history of your involvement with clinical budgeting.

Wickings: Okay, we've done a series of projects. The Westminster one was the first that I know of in which we did an experiment . . . and it certainly seemed to demonstrate some change. We could go into it if you're interested. . . . [Then at Brent] we tried to achieve the same changes just using costing data – I don't know how familiar you are with the distinctions and such like – we reported the cost to peer groups with various hypotheses about the high-cost group . . . and saw nothing for three years, despite everybody saying how valuable and important the information was. And so we then went into the Southend and Oldham and another district . . .

Researcher Two: East Birmingham?

Wickings: East Birmingham. And there we were trying to see whether one could get the same results using only the variable costs and excluding staffing and capital costs. . . . I get a bit irritated, people say, you know, 'You've been doing this for ten years, and what have you shown?' But in fact each time we've been trying a different approach and we believe that we've gradually learnt the conditions under which it's likely to be successful. We would no longer recommend it for universal adoption, certainly until some successful projects have run for a while, which hasn't happened yet . . .

Researcher Two: Is there a distinction between clinical budgeting and management budgeting?

Wickings: Well, there is yes, but it's a bit arcane. I mean I don't know how much detail you want to go into, but management budgeting – which is now called resource management – is concerned with the techniques of distributing costs to managers so that they can control them. . . . The differences are not all that clear. [In management budgeting] they also believed very much in charging out overheads. We did not in the projects that we've been engaged in, because we felt that it was important to emphasize those things the clinician could influence himself, you know . . .

Researcher One: I read the *Nuffield Portfolio*, there is an introduction from Tony Culyer, and he describes these clinical budgeting trials, or whatever, as experiments; I mean did you see it yourself as an experiment in that sense?

Wickings: Yes, I mean; yes we tried, in so far as we could, to set it up so that you would get genuine learning, so I suppose, I don't like the phrase 'experimenting', but yes, I don't mind, I suppose . . . we worked – sorry I'm sort of stammering really – we certainly saw it as being innovative, and therefore worthwhile if you were going to learn from it, of trying to establish some reasonable sorts of controls, you know and such like, it makes it more complicated and such like. And because of the difficulty of learning from these things and forming balanced judgements, there were various ways you ought to evaluate the project.

Researcher One: I noticed there was an Evaluation Group set up . . .

Wickings: That's right, and they think it's the best thing since fish-fingers more or less, they were very supportive. But you see that's an example that one of the difficulties we felt . . . was of defining what success is.

Researcher Two: Returning to the point about the experiment nature of it. I mean I got the impression when I read the beginning of this report [Wickings *et al.* 1985] these were being set up as kind of like *tests* of the idea, and something riding on these particular events . . .

Wickings: I think that's probably right, I mean there's a limited number of occasions on which you'll get governmental money to try things out . . .

Researcher Two (laughing): Sure.

Wickings (laughing): Precisely. Particularly if they're expensive as in many senses this was. I still think actually that it's a piddling little investment compared with the importance of trying to be able to get a negotiated set of expectations of what each expect of the other, from general managers and clinicians, but obviously you have to be very discreet. We thought it would be easier than it was. There were terrible difficulties due to the repeated reorganizations of the health service. I mean that genuinely, it meant that people were coming and going, and that people were without staff and so on and so forth.

Researcher One: This affected the Birmingham part of the study didn't it?

Wickings: It affected all of them. Birmingham was part of it, but it also affected Southend. At one stage, only the district administrator had been working in Southend out of *any* of the managers for longer than a year . . . and to expect them to be introducing new ways of working immediately during that period was very difficult. And there were three successive changes in Oldham, but I mean that's what the world's like I'm afraid, but it makes it very difficult; I often wished I was injecting rats in cages.

Researcher One: Could you make an argument that in a sense for a successful clinical budgeting system to work, you must be able to deal with those sort of . . .

Wickings: Yes, you're right . . . the period that you *don't* want people to go is when you're setting them up. You know, we never got to any sort of stage. . . . And I think we're going to find the same troubles with the resource management system; that it's very difficult to set it up. I think, going back to the point I was making, a lot depends on whether you have managers of the capacity to cope with it, who want to go on doing it. . . .

Researcher One: Your various economic criteria, there wasn't actually much change as I understand it in . . .

Wickings: Well, I don't regard those as a success, I don't think they demonstrated very much, except that in the circumstances in which we tried it, it didn't work.

Researcher One: Yeah, and you put something, I quote from the report: 'It sounds perverse to regard the experiments as encouraging rather than disappointing'.

Wickings: Yes.

Researcher One: So you regard the experiment, that those ones are largely a failure then?

Wickings: Well, I don't like these words 'failure' and 'success'. You know how these things work don't you?

Researcher One: Yes.

Wickings: What I meant, the things I felt that we could really be encouraged by, were that it was never rejected, firstly. We can try and start in a new system, and if you've worked with doctors very much – have you worked with clinicians in hospitals?

Researcher One: No.

Wickings: Well, they're an extremely powerful and rightly I think arrogant lot by and large, very independent, idiosyncratic, they're not managed by anybody you see, they're like professors. And, that to get them to accept changes of this sort is always difficult. Now, by and large, the medical staff were either apathetic, or supportive, there were one or two fierce opponents, but they were unusual. Where I felt the encouragement came was that if the managers had been able to do *their* bit, I think that the evidence was still encouraging – but obviously you can't be too unkind about people who've been very kind and worked for you over several years, I mean it's very good of them to have done it at all. . . . [For example] East Birmingham – the medical staff there, I hadn't, we had no problem with them at all, they were very keen. But I mean I stopped working there because the bloody DMT [District Management Team] weren't putting any effort into it, and you can't go on pouring money into these things unless people are putting some effort into it. I mean they were all different, you see one of the troubles, one was trying to do so many things at one time . . . we were testing out something to see whether it could be a national model – that was the idea. And our conclusions on that were, that you don't stand a hope in hell of doing it, if you haven't got at least some good models demonstrated by test pilots, that was the analogy we used.

Researcher One: Can I just go back to something in the report, the interim evaluation report which is attached to that appendix. . . . Would you say it's fairly positive?

Wickings: Yes, I mean I was, I was pleased. I think very correctly (*laughter*), I mean we felt that it was *our* job to present the results of our evaluation, and we couldn't ourselves claim that there was much evidence. Nonetheless, it's still our view that the potential of the system has not been invalidated at all, and that's what fortunately this Evaluation Group – they were quite tough with us at times – but they helped to say that there wasn't a better way forward in their view; that there is always going to be resource shortage, you have to find ways of handling that. That does in some way or another require some dealings between clinicians and managers, and although you haven't done it very well yet, that's the way forward, to do something like that.

Researcher Two: So in effect it wouldn't have mattered *what* the actual results were in the experimental districts.

Wickings: Yes it would, yes I think it would, I mean if there had been absolute confusion, I mean goodness knows what they would have said. But they didn't say – which was an expectation when we did our research originally – 'this should now be implemented nationally' (*bangs desk*). There was nothing like that. And what they really sanctioned was continued work to try and get it to work. And the resource management initiative is the same . . . and they're trying six districts with again different patterns, because it's bloody difficult.

Researcher One: That came through the Griffiths Report? The resource management?

Wickings: Yes, that's right.

Researcher One: Because that's one of the successes, Jim Blyth with the Griffiths commission.

Wickings: Well, Jim Blyth went down to see Southend . . . but you see again, I think he underestimated the complexity of it, because the Griffiths report said they had set these up to be implemented in six months. Well two years later they were just at the same stage we had been. It's much more complex than people seem to understand . . .

Researcher One: Why do you think people have underestimated the complexity of introducing this?

Wickings: It's partly the boredom factor. I mean, the health service is greedy for new ideas. And a new idea comes along, and everybody says, 'tremendous!' And for a while it's terribly fashionable, 'this is it!' and so on, and everybody assumes it's going to be working whisky-a-gogo in no time. . . . And then the actual business of setting that up and running it and bringing about social change in a very complex organization, everybody's found that – not just us, I mean you look at the literature about the introduction of social change in industry – to take a good many years to bring about a very complex change is as nothing. And from the outside, I mean I could have said to British Leyland: all they've got to do is have fewer people and produce more cars, and they'd be wonderful! That's what people think, but as you know when you try and do that *within* the organization, it's very difficult.

Researcher One: It's interesting the role of the researcher in this sort of dichotomy, because in a sense we researchers are always trying to stress how complicated it is, and it's difficult to get hard-and-fast findings. Well, in a sense the policy people say, 'well that's no use, no, we want to make these new policies'. Did you find yourself caught in that sort of dichotomy?

Wickings: Well, we were under a sort of pressure to produce results. I mean there wasn't any very great support for what you might call the delights of academic learning. They wanted results. But, I can certainly understand it. I think we all of course tend to see the things we're engaged in as more complex than others will see it unless they're involved in it. I don't know, I feel that the fact we were trying to change the model we were testing each time and that we were trying to bring about a very significant change in complex organizations at a time when the chief officers were regularly changing . . . I felt one shouldn't be discouraged by what one had seen, because there hadn't been any evidence to persuade one that it was wrong; that it was difficult, yes.

Researcher Two: But isn't it quite likely that given all this kind of turbulence, all these organizational changes being forced upon the health service, that people working within it and maybe especially consultants, would see the clinical budgeting effort, the PACTs experiments, as just another one of those? You know, another one in the train of . . .

Wickings: Yes. That's right. There's lots of people thinking that at the moment.

Researcher Two: I mean aren't they in a sense right, that it's just another one of those?

Wickings: Well yes, of course, it's just another one of those. It's not a sort of Holy Grail or anything like that. The health service has not been transformed by it. I mean it is now routinely accepted by most clinicians that they are going to have to work within a budget at some stage. . . . If you talk to the managers up and down the districts, they also feel that, that if the cash-limited state-funded system is going to be managed at all, it must be able to make choices: a bit more on this and less on that, and some sort of budgeting system is necessary for that. And I think, myself, that we were largely accountable for that change. The fact we haven't I'm afraid, been able to show it all working whisky-a-gogo is a pity, I wish we could, I'd be Sir Iden

Wickings or something now. (*Laughter.*) But that's how real life is, isn't it?

At this point coffee is brought in and the tape-recorder is switched off. Wickings asks the researchers whether this is the sort of thing they want from him because he has found the line of questioning rather unexpected. After reassurance from the researchers that the interview is working very well, Wickings goes on to outline the different forms of management budgeting and resource management which have been developed post-Griffiths. The interview resumes:

Researcher One: How do you judge success or failure in these resource management projects?

Wickings: I think that's very difficult. . . . The sorts of things that I would regard as being evidence of success, are that the people locally claim that they're able to be better social actors now than they were before, and can produce some evidence to support that. Now, it would be very nice to be able to say that, you know, the mortality rates have dropped or something, but the likelihood of that being shown is so slight, and one just has to accept that that's not there. What I would call constructive redeployment of funds is some evidence of it being useful I think, particularly if people say, 'we can now do this, and we could do that, and we couldn't have done this without that system'. And the sort of picture I have in my mind's eye, of success, would be there being a set of overall plans . . . a set of plans for each specialty in which the managers and the clinicians both feel they're working to achieve the same things. And success will be that they both know what successful is like, you know, and that seems to me to be an important sort of social goal of these efforts.

Researcher One: It's interesting, in that CASPE report, some of the criteria for judging the success early on were listed as being economic, I mean they're like economic measures and your most recent one is very much; you said 'social actors' . . . my eyes sort of lit up . . .

Wickings: I think . . . (*Laughs.*) Yeah, there isn't a monocular view of the world is there? I mean if you have got one, you're more a fool I think, and one should if possible try and get a sort of vectorial approach of various views. At least I think that. But I mean I quite often have economists on, working in CASPE . . . I think economists are – I've just reviewed a book by Gavin Mooney – I think economists have a very mechanistic view of life: a view that people are logical. And the expectations they have are based upon various logical hypotheses about reactions to different incentives and so on and so forth. Now, I don't think obviously they do have to accept that, in fact people are far less logical than that and make the most bizarre choices and often hold contradictory views. When you actually work with them you find that they're in some cognitive dissonance way having difficulty with trying to reconcile the greatly conflicting views . . . I mean economics is a very helpful way to analyse transactions between people, I'm very persuaded by it. I'm quite glad I didn't do a first degree in economics mind you, because people who work with me who did that, they often seem to me to be irritated that people don't actually seem to work the way that they bloody well should, you know. . . . I'm not sure whether the changes are gross enough to be seen in these big studies, and that's one of the problems about it. And that's why it may be that you need to do more studies about what's happening at the micro level within the organizations and see if, if you believe that's . . .

Researcher Two: You'll need sociologists for that. (*Laughs.*)

Wickings: Yes there's no choice in that.

Researcher Two: Okay. Suppose it was instituted as a national policy throughout, throughout the NHS . . .

Wickings: Which I actually think it will, oddly enough, despite all the difficulties, I think it will, because I think it's logical (*laughs*); that sounds illogical.

Researcher Two: Right okay, well *if* it was . . .

Wickings: But not before 1995 I would say so.

Researcher Two: Okay, so it's a very long term . . .

Wickings: I think it will gradually come yes. Sorry, I keep interrupting . . .

Researcher Two: Yes, you do it quite successfully, I've forgotten what I was going to say (*laughs*). This always happens.

Wickings: Yes, clinical budgeting.

Researcher Two: Yes thank you, yes, that's what we were talking about. Yes, so how would you envisage the difference in the health service, from a patient's point of view? I mean would there be fewer waiting lists for instance?

Wickings: I passionately believe that we ought to be giving our patients a better deal than we now are. Often they're getting a very good deal, but there are many times they're not, and we don't seem to have the mechanisms to handle that. And I know I'm talking long term, and I'm talking on the assumption that one has got something, something like a national system, so I'm making *huge* gigantic leaps you realize that. But if you imagine that most districts had something like this, and that the information was shared, not only would you be able to have people like me say, 'Well this is what I would expect us to see. Why are we only seeing that?' As new consultants appeared, you'd be able to spell out what you thought they were going to do. . . .

Researcher One: You said during the coffee break that you found our questions quite extraordinary. Why, by the way?

Wickings: I don't know really. I hadn't really expected that the discussion would go this sort of way. And also I'm wondering if you're going around a whole series of projects like this, how you're going to draw common things together from them. I find that interesting. Will we be able in the end to see something written?

Researcher One: Oh, I hope so.

Researcher Two: We've already written three papers.

Researcher One: Some of our stuff, we've already presented it to the Health Economists' Study Group.

Wickings: Yes, unfortunately, I'm not a member of the HESG because I'm not a health economist you see . . .

Act V: An evaluation meeting

The research on clinical budgeting has at long last come to an end. Researcher One has managed to interview a member of the DHSS Evaluation Group – the first member of the group he had approached had refused to talk on the record. The paper for Brunel University has also been delivered. The three researchers are now sitting in Researcher One's office at the University of York. They are talking over what they have achieved in the research.

Researcher Two: My feeling is the Wickings interview went quite well. He gave us a lot of his time and seemed to talk freely. He definitely produced a 'weak programme' version of clinical budgeting. He said that he didn't like us referring to his research projects as 'experiments' and he pointed out that it was very hard to say what success or failure meant – he preferred to talk about it as a 'learning process'. The role of the PACTs agreements seems to have been to provide a 'negotiating framework' to get more explicit discussion between clinicians and managers of their future plans. The direct route to change on economic grounds advocated in his article in the *Nuffield/York Portfolio* – change measurable by 'direct observation' in 'experiments' – was replaced by a rather different conception. This is not to say that Wickings implied that PACTs were totally ineffective, but rather that what impact they had was not produced by doctors, managers and nurses simply acting as individual economic calculators. At one point I even heard him hinting that the underlying problems of the NHS were sociological rather than economic.

Researcher One: Yes, I thought he was going to offer us both jobs when he said that! Great! I thought, at last a bit of consultancy. Seriously though, the experimental rhetoric did rather seem to vanish when we got talking. In the end his research turned out not to be 'science' in the sense of physics, but neither did it seem a piece of 'quick and dirty' policy research. Remember how he himself referred to what he was doing. He said he had been 'doing this for ten years', 'trying a different approach [each time] to try and see'; he described it as 'a learning process', 'to try and see the conditions under which it's likely to be successful'. The science-like aspects were reduced to 'trying to establish some reasonable sorts of controls' thus 'making it more complicated', and he talked much more about evaluating it in terms of 'balanced judgements', and 'things we could really be encouraged by'.

Researcher Three: The language of hypothesis-testing and experimentation, of cut-and-dried success and failure, certainly doesn't seem to do such research justice. Maybe dealing with the 'real world' requires the sort of research where you learn slowly over a long period of time by trial and error.

Researcher Two: Quite possibly. But the scientific rhetoric which was dominant in the CASPE report made its appearance in the interview nevertheless; though admittedly usually in response to our formulations. But he quickly adopted the alternative way of talking and indeed seemed rather unsure of himself when we asked him outright whether he regarded the thing as an experiment.

Researcher One: I know, but it only makes me depressed. I started off this project thinking we'd at last found some real science – 'forget your QALYs', I thought, 'it may not be physics, but at least they have experiments' – and it turns out that it dissolves into something which as far as I can see is not too dissimilar to sociology.

Researcher Two: And it's all the better for that too. I can't see why you're depressed at finding that out. I'm more reassured. And physics is not so different either – at least according to modern sociology of science.

Researcher Three: And if you weren't so obsessed with physics you would see that the sort of 'participant-centred' sensitive research which Wickings has evolved is probably the best that you can do in a policy context. You've got to admire him for having stuck with it for so long.

Researcher One: If you insist. But then we still have the problem that he isn't a proper health economist. Anyway, moving on, at least I got some real dirt from the member of the Evaluation Group I interviewed.[4] It turns out that the Group was under direct pressure from the government. I don't think either of you have seen the transcript yet. Perhaps I could read some of the relevant pieces to you?

Researcher Two: You managed to use the tape-recorder this time did you?

Researcher One: Sort of. I felt there might be problems after the first person we approached said he didn't want to talk on the record at all.

This time I managed to record half an interview. He let me use the recorder alright, but then we were interrupted by a phone call and – I'm embarrassed to say this – when I started the recorder again I pushed the wrong button. I'm really incompetent I'm afraid.

Researcher Two: That's why you never made it as a physicist.

Researcher One: I realized what had happened as soon as I had finished and I hastily wrote up some notes on the train back. Anyway (*shuffling through reams of papers on his desk*) here is the transcript and my notes (*producing several sheets of tatty typescript*). I started by asking him why they picked him for the Evaluation Group. He said he didn't have a clue. Right at the start he stressed the importance of the Evaluation Group being independent from Wickings's team. He said, 'The idea was that we would be independent of the groups that were actually involved in the process. So we weren't really part of the promotion activity. We were independent of it.' That's interesting because later on, as we'll see, he gives reasons as to why in fact they weren't actually independent. He then described the way the Group worked. They went out to visit the districts either alone or in pairs and tried to talk to everyone including the disaffected people who didn't think the thing was working. He was really quite proud that they had tried to find the disaffected people. Now here is the best bit, he's talking about the production of the report: 'Then we got to a point where they decided, they suddenly decided in my view too hurriedly that we were to report, a sudden decision that we were to report. And I know why that was taken because by that stage the Department, the government, had decided that they really wanted to move ahead on this, and they thought all this pithering around, this slow development was really a waste of time and energy. We had to make a big push and they wanted to know quickly what the lessons were from what we had done. They were also very dissatisfied with us as an Evaluation Group, obviously, that we were also pithering around.'

Researcher Two: So there was direct government pressure on the Evaluation Group. At what level did the pressure come?

Researcher One: That's what I asked him next and he said, 'Somebody high up the system'. He also says that after that they decided to do away with Evaluation Groups altogether. Anyway he said later that he felt most uncomfortable about the whole way of working and that it was this government chief scientist, Buller, the head of the Evaluation Group, who was orchestrating things.

Researcher Two: That's wonderful, a very clear example of direct external pressure on research, the sort of evidence which it is very difficult to get in sociology of science. A hard-and-fast case of political pressures directly impacting on how scientific facts are constructed.

Researcher One: Yes, I thought you would like that.

Researcher Three: Much as I dislike the present government, I feel slightly uneasy at the way you two are willing to accept this bit of interview data so uncritically. After all, it is only one version, and if we talked with Buller he might very well give a different account of what went on.

Researcher One: Come off it, that's taking this stuff on versions too far. It is just a fancy way of talking to avoid biting the real political bullet. It may be a version, but it is the one I would be prepared to put my money on.

Researcher Two: Yes, and what about your argument about the need to produce an appropriate version for the occasion at hand. Surely the relevant occasion in terms of our research has got to be the opportunity to deal with the politics of the NHS and to criticize Thatcher's policies. We can't hide behind some sort of bogus neutrality by saying it's all just a matter of versions.

Researcher Three: Well, I don't think we can resolve that issue here. Perhaps the final chapter of the book might be a more appropriate place for that. But getting back to your respondent – the evaluator – did he disagree with the conclusion the Evaluation Group produced?

Researcher One: Well, that's the problem. By and large he did agree.

Researcher Three: So you could argue that in this case the government's intervention simply speeded up the inevitable.

Researcher One: You could argue that, but I'm not going to. This evaluator has a rather frustrating attitude towards the success or failure of the clinical budgeting experiments. Like Wickings he spent most of his time outlining what was wrong and the horrendous problems they faced, but despite all that, he concludes that they're still the only way forward. Here, listen to this: 'I mean they know one or two things from it, for example, the system won't work without a high degree of commitment from management that they will change their managerial style to make it work. I mean I felt that there were far too many people who felt that this experiment was a sort of substitute for taking a tough management line, somehow clinical budgeting was going to solve the problem for you; it wasn't . . .'

Researcher Two (interrupting): That's an interesting argument. He seems to be saying that the experiment itself got in the way and adversely affected managers' practices – a kind of Heisenberg disturbance of the system with the measuring instrument.

Researcher One: I'm pleased to hear that you can use a bit of physics too. The point is, he goes on to be pretty scathing about the experience of PACTs: '. . . the clinicians, I mean some of them, they were more sceptical because they thought it was all a trick to get money out of them. They were right in their suspicion, which I think was one of the things that was really bad, and the management weren't strong enough to run the system . . .' But then having said all that he still came out in favour of it: 'Well I think we went through all the difficulties you see. And then one said, "Okay, well what are we saying? Are we saying it's all so difficult we should give up? Or are the difficulties there because it's fundamentally misconceived, or despite the difficulties we should soldier on?" It was at that point that we did come to the overall view that it wasn't misconceived. I mean it does have the right ingredients, and the question then is, is it worth struggling to make sure these ingredients are present and used in the right way? . . . Generally one has to struggle with it. I mean they had three goes and three failures but there was no reason to stop just yet.'

Researcher Two: What is the role of the test, then, if you go on struggling with it after the thing has failed?

Researcher One: Well, of course, I asked him that but he just went back to a priori grounds as to why it was so good: 'It has the elements in it that you think a good management system should have. The PACT – this is the central feature – the PACT is the focus of negotiation . . .' and so on.

Researcher Three: So his view of it is rather like Wickings's – it is all about providing a management structure or a context within which people can negotiate.

Researcher One: That's right. Unfortunately I can't be 100 per cent sure because the tape stopped then. But I did manage to record the bit where he had doubts about the independent status of the Evaluation Group: 'In a way I felt the Evaluation Group got too close to Iden Wickings. . . . We were almost pushed into a role of helping him design his system better by feeding back to him the criticisms that were given. . . . And I can see that in the interests of health service management that might be a good idea, but from the point of view of doing strict evaluation, I think we should have been more detached than we actually were. I think we got – I won't say captured because we are not easy people to capture . . .' When I suggested that maybe he was 'sucked' into it he replied, 'Well, we got pushed into a slightly different role. We got pushed into a role of helping the experiments to work, rather than evaluating them as they stood. . . . Well, that's fair enough, but I don't think it's quite what an Evaluation Group should be doing. But, on the other hand, I think it was better having us there than what they have done since. Which is to say without evaluation'.

Researcher Three: So even the evaluators seem to have ended up assisting the process of application – a kind of 'weak programme of evaluation', which contrasts strongly with your earlier quotation from this evaluator where he talked about the merits of independent evaluation.

Researcher One: That's right. So many of the interviews oscillate around this double rhetoric, where one moment everything is scientifically hunky dory, rigorous and independent, and the next it is all couched in vague phrases like 'better having us there than not' or 'helping the experiments to work', and so on. For instance, earlier in the interview the evaluator criticized other health service studies for not having proper evaluation and at that point he offered quite a different version of scientific method. I had asked for his reaction to the point that at the CERN particle accelerators they don't need evaluators and he replied, 'But they're doing experiments, aren't they? . . . It's more like, say, well we're going to experiment, with artificial insemination, and we're just going to do it, okay and then that's it. Well, and then the people who are involved can, if you care to ask them, they may give you their experiences of it, but I mean there is no attempt by any independent body to evaluate the experiment. It seems to me that is quite bad. . . . That's the sort of thing that is happening in the health service all the time. People are going off in this direction and going off in that direction, if they have a nice experience they talk about it, if they have a nasty experience they talk about it, but it is totally unsystematic.'

Researcher Two (ironically): Unlike his experience of evaluating the clinical budgeting experiments!

Researcher Three: There always seems to be a contrast made with some hypothetical group who are doing things worse in terms of some model of scientific method – in this case people having 'nice experiences' and 'nasty experiences' which they merely 'talk about', counterposed with systematic independent evaluation. This appears to be the way it always works: contrasting pairs of opposed versions of scientific method, either to deconstruct an overly systematic version, as Wickings did to economics in his interview, by saying it is too mechanistic, inflexible and simplistic, and doesn't take account of real social actors or whatever; or more usually to deconstruct soft research by saying it isn't hard, rigorous, tested with independent evaluation, or whatever. Anyway, I'm curious to know how you got on at Brunel. That must have been difficult: an audience of general sociologists, sociologists of science and all sorts of economists – and all at once.[5]

Researcher One: I was trying to forget about that. That was another depressing experience. I gave the paper which dealt with all that stuff about clinical budgeting being a social technology – you know, an attempt to change human behaviour with the use of economics – and which treated the CASPE experiments as a test of this social technology. Then I went on to deconstruct the tests in the way I've talked about before, by a little analysis of CASPE report, which showed what a disaster they had actually been. I read out the list of the so-called 'points of encouragement' resulting from the tests and there were just howls of laughter from the audience, especially when I came to the bit about the ward sisters enjoying being budget holders. But then I got pulled apart in an odd kind of way in the question session, or rather pulled in several directions at the same time. No one seemed entirely happy with what I had done. In the first place, a sociologist interested in macrosociology said that it was clear that the whole thing was really to do with the role of the state and Thatcher's policy to squeeze the NHS and my study didn't tell us enough about this wider context in which the experiments were taking place. Then there was a sociologist of science who argued against this macro-sociologist but who was also dismissive of my paper because he said everyone knew economics wasn't a proper science, and so what? Then one of the economists, who seemed to be something of a theorist, got uptight with the sociologists for saying that economics was just a matter of social contingency; he felt there was more to proper economics than that, and in a way I was in sympathy with this view because of course I wanted to show that there was something worth deconstructing in the first place. Finally, there was this health economist and he said that of course clinical budgeting experiments were nothing to do with economics, but then he said he had just been given a contract by the DHSS to evaluate the latest resource management experiments! (*Speaking in an increasingly garbled fashion.*) So there I was trying first of all to argue against the macrosociologist by pointing out to her that the wider social context such as Thatcherism only took on meaning in people's everyday practices, such as their experiences with these experiments, so of course I sided with the sociologist of science who supported me on this, but then found myself arguing against him by saying that economics was the social science most in need of deconstruction and hence ended up agreeing with the uptight economic theorist; then I proceeded to argue against the health economist who claimed clinical budgeting wasn't health economics at all by saying that it must be health economics because everyone working in health economics including himself always said that real health economics was what other people did, ha ha – and anyway why was he evaluating the resource management experiments if they weren't health economics? By the way, I said I would send him the final version of our study in case it was of any use to him in his evaluation.

Researcher Two: Poor guy!

Researcher Three: Anyway, you survived. It sounds to me as if you did the usual bits of juggling which people have to do to survive in the social world: for each successive practical occasion constructing and deconstructing agreements and alliances by constructing and deconstructing versions of sociology and economics as you go along. Of course, normally it isn't such hard work because you don't get all these different groups with all their different versions together in one place.

Researcher One: Except, perhaps, in the health service.

Researcher Two: It seems to me that we ought to get clear just what it is that is inadequate about the Brunel version of clinical budgeting.

Researcher One: There's no problem there. What was wrong was that I took only one version of clinical budgeting – the strong programme version – and deconstructed it by recovering the weak version.

Researcher Two: That's not quite how I see it. I think what you did was to privilege the strong version of success, as formulated in Wickings's scientific rhetoric, by using *that* to deconstruct the weak version of success – the ward sisters enjoying their budgets, and so on. By doing so, you effectively offered your own evaluation of the results of the experiments: they were a failure and not, as the Evaluation Group and the ward sisters and Wickings in his sociological mood all thought, a (qualified) success. In short, far from using the weak-programme version of clinical budgeting to deconstruct the strong-programme version, as you claimed just now, I think you did the exact opposite: you deconstructed the weak version with the strong version.

Researcher One: You may be right. In any case, we clearly need to think hard about how we are going to write this stuff up for the book. But I'm worried that if we give equal prominence to both versions – *à la* BBC – we'll end up not really saying anything.

Researcher Three: Alternatively, like the health economists, we could choose to present the version which is most suitable for the practical occasion at hand.

Researcher One: Whatever that might be!

Researcher Two: In that case we've got to make up our minds what the practical occasion is. I mean, are we doing real science, or 'quick and dirty' policy research, or sensitive participant-centred research?

Researcher One: We don't want to spend years on this, so we can't be doing that last one. And we're not getting paid enough and have already taken too much time to be doing a 'quick and dirty', and we're too incompetent to be doing science. Perhaps we can leave what it is we *are* doing until the conclusion.

Researcher Two: That doesn't give us much breathing space. There's only one more chapter before we get there.

Researcher Three: Right. So let's think about this carefully . . .

Notes

1. All the excerpts quoted here are taken from a talk given at a course for senior

clinicians entitled 'Effectiveness and Efficiency in Patient Care: A Seminar for Clinicians' held at Bowness-on-Windermere, Cumbria, England on 17–18 March 1986.

2. Quotations from 'Kathleen' and from Peter West are taken from a transcript of the HESG meeting, University of Bath, 7 July 1986.
3. The interview with Iden Wickings was conducted on 2 February 1987.
4. The interview with the evaluator took place on 11 March 1988.
5. One of us (Pinch) delivered a paper entitled 'Clinical Budgeting in the NHS: The Testing of a Social Technology' to the Centre for Research into Innovation, Culture and Technology (CRICT), 9 March 1988.

7 The rationalized choice: option appraisal and the politics of rational decision-making

> A major element in appraisal is its explicitness. The logic of a decision has to be apparent.
>
> (Akehurst 1987: 22)

> Now, what you're trying to do is to get numbers to work for you, trying to get numbers to reflect your value judgements. And it's important never to lose sight of that. The numbers have got to be your servant.[1]

Politics, appraisal and the politics of appraisal

The two techniques for reforming health care provision we have examined so far – outcome measurement by means of QALYs (Ch. 5) and clinical budgeting schemes (Ch. 6) – are in fairly early stages of development, acceptance and implementation. While both of these, at least to most health economists, promise major improvements in the efficiency of the health care system, it would be difficult to claim that they have as yet had much impact on the practical performance of the NHS. In contrast, the procedure of option appraisal, which is our topic in this chapter, is a relatively well-established technique both in terms of its theoretical and technical pedigree and its degree of embeddedness within the current practices of the NHS.

C.B.A

Option appraisal, as a type of economic analysis, is one of the family of techniques which follow what health economists call the cost–benefit approach. Other members of the family include investment appraisal, cost–effectiveness analysis, cost–utility analysis and cost–benefit analysis (Culyer 1985b: 3). In principle, the technique of appraising prospective ways of doing something by identifying and valuing their benefits and their costs in order to determine the option with the best value for money may be used as a completely general planning tool.

Within the contexts of health economics and health service administration, however, the term 'option appraisal' usually refers to the use of cost–benefit evaluation in the planning of service developments which involve major capital spending such as the building of a new hospital or the rationalization of the current provision of resources.

Since 1981, option appraisals have been mandatory within the NHS in England and Wales for the spending of capital sums of over £5 million (DHSS 1981a). District and/or Regional Health Authorities are obliged to carry out a detailed cost–benefit appraisal of various different ways of meeting the required service objectives and then to submit the results to the DHSS for 'Approval in Principle' (AIP). Without AIP, the spending cannot go ahead. Moreover, since 1982 option appraisals have been required even for those plans not expensive enough to involve Departmental approval. Health economists working in universities are frequently employed as consultants to the Health Authority planning teams involved in carrying out these procedures. However, because the option appraisal process is initiated and carried out as a practical task within the NHS rather than as a piece of academic research, examples have seldom been published. Those which have include Akehurst (1986), Akehurst and Holtermann (1985), Henderson, McGuire and Parkin (1984a, 1984b), Henderson *et al.* (1985), West, Mooney and Trevillion (1984) and Yule and Cohen (1985). All of these are discussion papers rather than peer-reviewed articles, and all make clear their orientation towards potential NHS option appraisers rather then fellow academic health economists. In short, they are published as teaching materials rather than research findings.

In addition to this 'worked example' literature, is a set of publications which offer generalized guidelines, handy hints and tips.[2] There is also a series of texts which review and survey the prospects and practices of option appraisal as it is currently carried out.[3] These texts are the most explicit on the benefits to be had from 'decision-making that embraces option appraisal enthusiastically and wholeheartedly' (Mooney and Henderson 1984: 14). Many of these texts employ the strategy of argumentation in which the perceived deficiencies of the 'usual' procedures for planning new service developments involving capital spending are contrasted with the efficiency-enhancing, rationality-producing procedure of appraisal (see Ch. 2 for a detailed examination of this form of argument). Option appraisal is seen as enhancing the rationality of NHS decision-making which, in its absence, is taken to suffer from the irrational effects of politics. Thus, while important decisions have of course been made without the benefit of appraisal, 'the challenge to the policy-makers appears to have been more about placating competing health service interests than promoting health interests, more about keeping the system well oiled than well directed and more about coping with the consequences than probing into the problems' (Mooney and Henderson 1984: 14).

Option appraisal is portrayed as rational, systematic, explicit and objective; it clearly promises to improve the quality of NHS decision-making for the benefit of everybody. However, this 'strong-programme rhetoric' (see Chs. 2 and 6) is usually modified in two main ways. First, care is taken to correct any impression that option appraisal is a mechanistic *substitute* for decision-making and the operation of skilled and experienced judgement:

> It can only be an aid to decision making, not a substitute for it.
> (Ludbrook and Mooney 1984: 3)

> Appraisal is not a substitute for judgement – but it should clearly indicate the important judgements that have to be made.
> (Akehurst and Buxton 1985: 6)

> The task of . . . appraisal is to make explicit the factors which impinge on the choice of option but it should never be viewed as a substitute for explicit decision-making
> (West, Mooney and Trevillion 1984: 26)

Second, some authors recognize that the perceived defects of NHS planning practices constitute the *environment* in which the option appraisal process must operate. That is, the very practices which appraisal is designed to change stand as obstacles to the successful operation of the change-making procedure itself.

> The spirit of appraisal must . . . not be at odds with the environment within which it is used. Its rational principles must not be devalued by arbitrariness. Its logical consequences must not be frustrated by unnecessary constraints in the NHS 'management system'.
> (Akehurst and Buxton 1985: 6)

The devaluation and frustration of the spirit of appraisal may be caused by Politics:

> Those with powerful political allies or who know how to manipulate public opinion [see Ch. 4] may be able to push decision makers to choose an option which on more rational grounds would not be preferred.
> (Mooney and Henderson 1984: 21)

Alternatively, it could happen in a more subtle way, as in the following 'charade account' given in interview by an insider (see also Ch. 3, 3.17):

> *Insider:* There is this sort of political – in the little 'p' – organizational sort of structure that's in there: the charade as it were of

an option appraisal will be used to present an argument which is the one that people want anyway, right? So it's like dressing it up in such a way that . . .

Interviewer: You feel you're going to get some added credence do you?

Insider: Well that's it. I mean you've gone through the motions, and I mean no one can argue with you, there it is, it's an option appraisal you know, and it's telling you exactly what it is that everyone wanted in the first place.

In all these accounts by health economists the rationality, explicitness and systematicity of the process of option appraisal is contrasted with the irrational, hidden and arbitrary procedures of other forms of health service planning. Their basic structure is appraisal versus politics. And while it is recognized that appraisal has to operate in a political – as well as a Political – context, the hope and expectation is that, if it can avoid political contamination, appraisal can *replace* politics as a decision-making procedure.

One of the major types of decision to which option appraisal is said to be most applicable is that of a rationalization of capacity. This is not simply because such decisions usually involve relatively large expenditures but because, particularly in the case of recent plans to rationalize acute services, they take place 'against the background of various government pronouncements about increased priority for other services [and other] pressures for rationalization' (Mooney and Henderson 1984: 8).

> The political issues loom large here as they always do when an attempt is made to close any NHS facility. It is in just such circumstances that option appraisal can provide a useful, systematic approach to planning.
>
> (ibid.: 8)

Interestingly, the structure of this argument is similar to the 'charade account' given above. What is 'useful' about an option appraisal in both cases is that it provides an effective means of justification for a decision taken for reasons external to the appraisal itself. In both cases, the appraisal enhances the credibility of a decision taken with its aid and increases the 'opportunity cost' entailed in opposing it (see Latour and Woolgar 1979). The difference between these two accounts is in the legitimacy of the role that 'politics' is perceived to play. In the case of the 'charade account', politics is that which illegitimately subverts the spirit of appraisal. In Mooney and Henderson's 'rationalization account', however, politics plays two roles. It both provides the (legitimate) 'background' in the form of 'pronouncements' and 'pressures' and also appears as the (illegitimate) 'political issues' attendant on attempts to close facilities. Here, option appraisal can be understood as a directly political tool used to justify decisions taken in line with the former kind of politics and to counteract opposition to those same decisions animated by the latter kind.

Three of the six published option appraisals cited above were connected with rationalization decisions (West, Mooney and Trevillion 1984; Akehurst 1986; Henderson, McGuire and Parkin 1984a, 1984b [both of these papers report on the one appraisal]). This context is made very clear in the title of Akehurst's paper, *Planning Hospital Services: An Option Appraisal of a Major Health Service Rationalisation*. We will now examine this paper in some detail.

Our focus, however, is not so much on the politics of health service rationalization as on the politics of economic rationality exemplified in the textual rendering of this particular appraisal. Nevertheless, the 'background' of the health authority's need to rationalize services and the 'political issues' of potential opposition to the decision are never far from the surface. If we ourselves appear to be backgrounding such important real-worldly concerns in favour of our detailed analysis of numerical and verbal argument, the reader should, in all charity, remember that it is in these esoteric details that the logic and the persuasive power of the option appraisal lies.

Reading *Planning Hospital Services*

We have chosen *Planning Hospital Services* (PHS – Akehurst 1986) for examination because it is by far the most detailed and explicit of the set of published appraisals. As we have mentioned, it is concerned with an important and large-scale decision taken in the highly political context of a rationalization of services. Furthermore, it is the only one of these appraisals to take the form (or very nearly, as we will see) of an Approval in Principle (AIP) document. The importance of this last point is that AIPs necessarily document *decisions*. The tension, which we noted above, in the option appraisal literature on the precise role of appraisals in the decision-making process is most clearly manifest in a text in which both an appraisal and the particular decision to which it contributed are documented. Thus we concentrate in the analysis on the results of the appraisal and particularly the final choice which emerged from the process.

The rationale for publishing PHS was stated by the author in his Preface as follows:

> The preparation of Approval in Principle submissions is likely to be a once in a lifetime event for most health districts and is a rare event even for some regions. In consequence, many officers find preparing the major part of the submission, the Option Appraisal,

> to be an unfamiliar and daunting task. The guidance material written by the Treasury and the DHSS, while helpful, is not detailed enough to sort out many of the problems which arise. In these circumstances knowledge of how previous appraisals have been conducted can save much time and effort, and it is for this reason that this Discussion Paper has been published.
>
> (Akehurst 1986: Preface)

Our approach to this text is guided by the author's claims in the Preface for the status and utility of the publication. In the quotation above we are told that reading PHS will provide us with 'knowledge of how previous appraisals have been conducted'. This is because PHS consists of the original report of an actual appraisal conducted by a planning team to which the author acted as consultant and report writer. PHS differs from the original report in at least three respects. First, it includes two pages of extra annotations (including the Preface) in order to provide 'some background . . . on the reasons why steps were taken in the way they were, and the process involved'. Second, eight of the original thirteen appendices are omitted 'where what they would contain is obvious'. Finally, the district and the hospitals involved are given 'fictitious' names. Essentially, then, PHS is designed to allow the reader public access to the most significant parts of a private report.

However, the fact that all that is needed to achieve this change in status are the minor alterations mentioned above suggests something about the kind of text represented by the original report. As stated in the Preface, the 'Approval in Principle document was meant to stand alone in the sense that anyone picking it up should be able to understand the reasoning processes described therein'. In other words, the original report was itself designed as a 'public' text in the sense that it should contain within itself everything needed to make a judgement as to the adequacy of the conclusions arrived at. A recent *AIP Bulletin* issued by the DHSS makes just this point about the presentation of AIPs: 'An AIP should be a self-contained document. . . . It should be capable of being read by a lay reader, taking them logically through [the steps of analysis] and thereby to the selection of the preferred option' (DHSS 1987b: 5). It appears that the desired explicitness and systematicity of the appraisal *as a process* is here translated into the textual quality of self-containedness, or independence. Sufficient unto itself, the ideal option appraisal should be self-explanatory. The lay reader, in order to understand its logic and its practical recommendations, should not need to consult other texts. However, given a lay reader as persistent as we have been, who *really* wishes to find out what *really* went on, the claim for textual independence begins to look rather fragile, as does the claim for the explicitness and rationality of the procedure itself.

Before we address such matters, we must describe the setting for the appraisal and, briefly, how it proceeded. The appraisal concerns the rationalization of hospital services, currently provided at five sites (Crompton General, Southside, Northside, Stones and Gordon's hospitals) within the Crompton District Health Authority; 'a district . . . characterised by severe problems of social deprivation with associated high mortality and morbidity' (Akehurst 1986: 4). The *problem* for the planning team was a tricky one: how best 'in line with Regional policy . . . to achieve substantial reductions in beds and revenue expenditure [i.e. running costs] by 1993' (ibid.: 4). The solution arrived at is to exchange quantity for quality, and to spend capital monies in order to save revenue expenditure: 'Capital developments will facilitate the achievement of these revenue savings as well as correcting deficiencies in services' (ibid.: 4). The *objectives* for the appraisal 'followed naturally' (ibid.: 18) from the policy of expenditure reduction on the one hand and the desire to improve services on the other. Six major objectives were arrived at:

A. Release revenue
B. Improve services to the elderly
C. Improve acute services
D. Improve Regional Specialty provision located in the District
E. Improve Accident and Emergency [A and E] facilities
F. Improve out-patient services[4] (ibid.: 4)

An additional four considerations provided further criteria by which options were compared:

G. Acceptability
H. Ease of staffing
I. Accessibility
J. Overall flexibility (ibid.: 21)

Initially, a total of 208 discrete 'options' were generated. An option is an operationalization of the set of objectives; that is, any configuration of services and sites that is considered capable of meeting the objectives. The next stage was the reduction of this long list of options to a short list to be assessed in detail. This was done by the imposition of a set of agreed constraints such as minimum standards of service (ibid.: 22–4). The short list consisted of six options which were then evaluated in detail. One of these six was a so-called 'do nothing' option, which involved little or no capital expenditure and which was assumed to be able to achieve the required service reduction by other means. Two separate forms of assessment were undertaken on all six options. Assessment of *cost* entailed calculating the estimated capital and revenue expenditures and then by taking into account the different time periods and lifespans of the developments proposed in each option arriving at a figure representing each option's annual equivalent cost (AEC). Assessment of *benefit* consisted of scoring each option – on a scale of 1 to 10 where 10 is optimal – on each relevant non-financial criterion (i.e. objectives B–E and G–J above) and then assigning each criterion a weight according to its importance relative to the others, the sum of the weights being designed to equal 100. The weight was then multiplied by the score to give an indication of the expected performance of each option on each criterion. Finally, all the weighted scores accruing to an option were added together to give that option's benefit score (see Table 7.4 below).

The final choice

The final stage in the assessment of the options' relative performance was to bring the separate cost and benefit components together as in Table 7.1, which is from the summary. From these results the preferred option was selected. It is of course . . .

From an inspection of Table 7.1 alone, it is not possible to select a 'clear winner'. This is because the process of appraisal has failed to produce an option which is superior to all the others, that is one which possesses the joint characteristics of lowest cost and highest benefit. In the absence of such an option one can attempt to attack the problem from the other direction. That is, one can look for a 'clear loser' – the option with the highest cost and lowest benefit – and reject it (Henderson 1984: 23). By repeating this process the choice may be narrowed down. Unfortunately, just as there is no option which is clearly superior, there is no clearly inferior one either.

So how was the selection made? Here is the first sentence of the explanation as given in the summary (Akehurst 1986: 5): 'Option 6 (Do Nothing) has been rejected because of its unacceptably low benefit

Table 7.1 The results

	Annual equivalent cost of capital and revenue together (£000s)	*Benefit score*
Option 1	38,425	702
Option 2	38,534	707
Option 3	38,600	688
Option 4	38,815	469
Option 5	38,559	675
'Do Nothing'	38,185	322

Source: Akehurst 1986: 5.

score.' With the removal of Option 6, to which we return below, the choice becomes less intractable. We can now reject Option 4 because it has the highest cost and lowest benefit of the remaining options. This leaves us with Options 1, 2, 3 and 5. We can now apply the rule of superiority/inferiority (or 'dominance' [Akehurst 1987: 9]) to select the first *pair* of these options (1 and 2) in preference to the second (3 and 5). The final choice, then, is between Options 1 and 2. It is here that the selection rules we have been using break down. To dramatize the nature of the choice between Option 1 and Option 2, here are two symmetrical explanations, each of which *might* have been given, but only one of which *was* (Akehurst 1986: 5):

Option 1: Option 6 (Do Nothing) has been rejected because of its unacceptably low benefit score. Option 1 has been selected as the preferred solution because it is the cheapest of the remaining options and has a benefit score close to the highest.

Option 2: Option 6 (Do Nothing) has been rejected because of its unacceptably low benefit score. Option 2 has been selected as the preferred solution because it has the highest benefit score of the remaining options and is close to the cheapest.

The final choice was Option 1.

If this summary of the explanation was all we had to go on, the selection of Option 1 rather than Option 2 might suggest, other things being roughly equal, that in the trade-off between the importance of (low) cost on the one hand and (high) benefit on the other, it is cost that was the preferred criterion. However, when we turn to the main text, an alternative reason is given for selecting Option 1 in preference to Option 2. The stated reason for the choice is based on an assessment of the differences in magnitude between the two options' cost figures, on the one hand, and their benefit scores on the other:

> An examination of the remaining options [1–5] shows that on non-financial criteria [i.e. benefit score] option 2 is *slightly* superior to option 1, but it is *considerably* more expensive in both capital and revenue costs.
>
> (ibid.: 48; our emphases)

Based on the figures given in Table 7.1, this means that its five extra benefit points makes Option 2 'slightly superior' whereas its extra cost of £109,000 makes it 'considerably more expensive'.

This contrast between 'slightly' and 'considerably' does the considerable rhetorical work of making what might otherwise seem a qualitative choice between 'cost' and 'benefit' seem a quantitative choice between larger and smaller magnitudes. It is interesting that a verbal form of measurement rather than a numerical one is chosen to settle the issue. Up to this point, the text displays a cumulative process of translation from the verbal to the numerical culminating in Table 7.1. However, it *is* possible to use numbers rather than words at this juncture. (Of course, there is more than one way of doing so, just as there are alternative formulations to 'slightly' and 'considerably'.) We chose to measure the differences between £38,425,000 and £38,534,000 on the one hand, and 702 and 707 benefit points on the other, by expressing them in terms of the percentage increase of the larger numbers over the smaller. After borrowing a calculator, we came up with these figures: the difference in cost (AEC), described in the text as 'considerable', is 0.28 per cent; the difference in benefit score, described in the text as 'slight', is 0.71 per cent.

It is possible that we have misread the text here. The above (cost) calculation is based on a reading of the phrase 'in both capital and revenue costs' (ibid.: 48) as referring to the *combination* of these two costs as expressed by the total AEC. (In Table 7.1, total AEC is explained as 'capital and revenue together'.) However, if we read the phrase as

Table 7.2 Overall comparison of options

		Options					
Row	*£000s*	*1*	*2*	*3*	*4*	*5*	*Do nothing*
A	Capital cost (minus sales)	11,800	11,478	17,156	9,844	13,009	488
B	Revenue cost in 'steady state'	36,854	37,062	36,804	37,470	36,943	37,160
C	Saving of revenue relative to status quo	3,809	3,601	3,859	3,193	3,720	3,503
D	Efficiency saving included in revenue savings	306	98	356	+310*	217	–
E	Total 'annual equivalent cost'	38,425	38,534	38,600	38,815	38,559	38,185
F	Scores on non-financial criteria	702	707	688	469	675	322

* decreased efficiency.
Source: Adapted from Akehurst 1986: 47.

indicating the results of two distinct comparisons – *capital* with benefit, and also *revenue* with benefit – then the problems with the given grounds for the selection of Option 1 increase.

According to Table 7.2, the capital costs (row A) of Option 2 (£11,478,000) are £322,000 *less* than the capital costs of Option 1 (£11,800,000). And while the revenue costs (row B) are indeed greater for Option 2 (£37,062,000) than for Option 1 (£36,854,000), the significance of the magnitude of this difference is far from clear. If we carry out our percentage increase calculations on these figures, the difference is 0.56 per cent. So is this big or is this small? The question becomes even more difficult to answer once we take into account the caveat furnished in PHS:

> It should be noted that the differences in revenue costs [row B] are small in general, and errors in estimation would account for a good part of the differences. In addition, the differences are very small in comparison to the total savings in revenue [row C] that all options would be expected to achieve in their 'steady state'.
>
> (ibid.: 47–8)

If we compare this general declaration of 'small' differences with the specific claim for a 'considerable' difference between the relevant costs of Options 1 and 2, we think we have a warrant for looking in more detail at the particular numbers upon which the choice of Option 1 was based.

Which costs?

In attempting to understand the cost figures used in PHS the problem is not a lack of information. On the contrary, PHS is replete with costing data including twenty-one pages of appendices. Indeed, it is this very profusion which causes the problem. Elsewhere, we have described the various cost figures and their relationships in more detail (Ashmore, Pinch and Mulkay 1987). For present purposes we will compare just two sets of costs, both of which despite having the same label – 'total AEC' – differ in an interesting and unexplained manner (Table 7.3).

The set of cost figures on the left of Table 7.3 are the ones given in Tables 7.1 (ibid.: 5) and 7.2 (ibid.: 47). They also appear in a third table in the text (ibid.: 40). The other set of cost figures appear in a fourth table captioned 'Summary of costs' (ibid.: 74) which appears in an appendix on capital costs. It can be noticed that not only are the total costs for all options considerably (or slightly) larger in the second set than in the first but also that the rank ordering of the options is different. That the final choice seems to be between Options 1 and 2 is partly dependent on their being taken as the two cheapest remaining options

Table 7.3 Some differences in total costs

Options	*The figures from PHS: 5, 40, 47*		*The figures from PHS: 74*		
	Total AEC (£000s)	*Rank order (1 is cheapest)*	*Total AEC (£000s)*	*Rank order (1 is cheapest)*	*The differences between the figures (£000s)*
1	38,425	2	38,518	2	93
2	38,534	3	38,680	4	146
3	38,600	5	38,695	5	95
4	38,815	6	38,886	6	71
5	38,559	4	38,648	3	89
6	38,185	1	38,268	1	83

after the rejection of the 'do nothing' Option 6. If the second set of cost figures had been the ones inscribed in the choice, it is possible that Option 2, despite having the highest benefit score, would not have been 'in the frame' at all. According to these figures, the option nearest to Option 1 in terms of cheapness is Option 5. As this latter option has a relatively low benefit score, we think it likely that Option 1 would, in these circumstances, have been chosen with even greater alacrity.

However, if we take into consideration the numbers in the right hand column of Table 7.3, which are our calculations of the differences between the pair of total costs for each option, it seems that all is not lost for supporters of Option 2. The interesting thing about these figures is their variation; and particularly the variation between the figure for Option 2 and those for all the other options. The figure of £146,000 seems disproportionately large in comparison to the others. Indeed, the variance between the highest and the next highest figures (£146,000 and £95,000) is, at £51,000, more than double that between the second highest and lowest (£95,000 – £71,000 = £24,000). Our close examination shows that these discrepancies in AEC are themselves due to unexplained variations in revenue costs. It is clear that they could have had a major impact on the fortunes of Option 2.

Happily, the second set of total cost figures was evidently not used in the choice. Indeed, it would seem reasonable for the lay reader of PHS to discount this particular set of figures altogether as it appears once only, in an appendix, and without comment, whereas the other set appears in the opening summary, is presented on two further occasions, and is the object of considerable comment. Thus, by the commonsense reading strategy of 'triangulation within the text', we appear to have sufficient warrant to accept the latter set and reject the former. However reasonable this move may be, it is of course far from conclusive. But as lay readers of a self-contained text, it would seem the best we can do.

Numbers, anomalies and benefit scores

Option appraisal, as an analytical technique, depends for its credibility on a rhetoric of measurement and quantification. While not aspiring to the ideal of true cost–benefit analysis in which everything on both sides of the cost–benefit equation is rendered in monetary units (Williams 1972), the assessment of potential benefit, as well as of likely cost, is done by translating 'soft' judgements into 'hard' numbers. The technical point of such a procedure, of course, is to permit a range of complex comparisons to be carried out with relative ease. A more practical aim is to produce a consensus on the adequacy of the outcome among, at the very least, those who have taken part in an appraisal. Because their judgements will, ideally, have been taken into account by being incorporated into a number, and because the manipulation of numbers is famously 'explicit and systematic' the subsequent career of these judgements and their role in the final outcome can be seen to be 'objective and rational'. Even if one disagrees with the result of this process, it is difficult to argue against it. If the choice generated by an appraisal seems, to those involved, to be entirely counter-intuitive, this may itself be taken as an indication of the validity of the exercise: clearly, if nobody expected or wanted the result, the appraisal cannot have been conducted illegitimately to dress up a prior choice. (Accounts of the consensus-producing function of appraisals are given in Ch. 3, 3.17 and 3.23.)

The following discussion is concerned with some of the problems of benefit measurement as encountered in PHS. Even in the abstract, this procedure frequently is perceived as problematic. As Mooney and Henderson colourfully put it, 'benefit measurement remains the health economist's dream and the administrator's nightmare' (Mooney and Henderson 1984: 25). The numerical matrix of benefit scores is presented in Table 7.4. We have described above the basic procedures used in its production. Table 7.5 is a selection of the summarized assessments from which the numbers are derived.

Following on from our discussion of the anomalous set of 'total AEC' figures to be found in PHS, we will examine the four further 'anomalies' labelled as such in Tables 7.4 and 7.5. An 'anomaly' is our term for something encountered in the course of reading which appears to be inconsistent either with other components of the text or with more generally available criteria of textual adequacy. A lay reader's term would be, for example, 'error' or 'mistake'. During the course of our close reading of PHS we came upon nearly twenty such phenomena. (For a complete listing and analysis, see Ashmore, Pinch and Mulkay 1987.) These varied in significance from the clearly trivial case of the 'spelling mistake' or 'typing error' to those we examine here, the

Table 7.4 The benefit score matrix: numerical version

Objectives	*Options*						
	WT	*1*	2	3	4	5	Do *nothing*
Services to the elderly	25	8 (200)	6 (175) [*Anomaly* 4]	9 (225)	7 (175)	6 (150)	5 (125)
Acute services	22	6 (132)	8 (176)	7 (154)	2 (44)	7 (154)	1 (22)
Regional specialty	9	6 (54)	3 (27)	6 (54)	3 (27)	9 (81)	3 (27)
A & E	13	8 (104)	9 (117)	9 (117)	4 (52)	9 (117)	1 (22) [*Anomaly 1*]
Ease of staffing	9	1 (9)	6 (54)	7 (63)	7 (63)	4 (36)	7 (63) [*Anomaly* 2]
Accessibility	9	7 (63)	7 (63)	3 (27)	8 (72)	6 (54)	8 (72)
Accept-ability	9	7 (63)	6 (54)	4 (36)	3 (27)	4 (36)	1 (9)
Flexibility	4	8 (32) [*Anomaly* 3]	8 (32)	3 (12)	9 (36)	5 (20)	9 (36)
Total weighted score (out of 1,000)		702 [Resolution 3: −12 690]	707 [Resolution 4A: 0 707 or 4B: −25 682]	688	469	675	322 [Resolution 1: −9 313] [Resolution 2: +54 367]

Note: We have added the relevant anomalies and their calculated resolutions (see text for details) in square brackets.
Source: Adapted from Akehurst 1986: 46.

resolution of which has the effect of altering some of the given benefit scores.

Anomaly 1 has to do with the score for A and E (accident and emergency) provision given to Option 6. According to Table 7.4 the weighting for A and E is 13, while the score achieved by Option 6 for this

Table 7.5 Selections from the benefit score matrix: verbal version

Objectives	*Options*					
	1	2	3	4	5	6 *Do nothing*
Ease of staffing	[Score: 6	7	7	4	7	1]
	Single specialty hospital difficult to staff with paramedics Possible difficulties with medical staffing	Possibly difficulties over paramedics	Ideal on staffing acute beds Single specialty hospital difficult for paramedics	Four-site solution may cause problems with both medical staff and paramedics	Two geriatric day hospitals may lead to problems with para-medical staffing	As 2 [*Anomaly* 2]
Flexibility	[Score: 8	8	3	9	5	9]
The main flexibility issues relate to infectious diseases and geriatrics. For the latter, the fewer the sites, the less flexibility there is if norms increase. For ID, Southside is the most flexible and CGH the least.	Moder-ately flexible for geriatrics Most flexible for ID [*Anomaly* 3] [ID located: CGH	As 1 for geriatrics As 1 for ID Southside	Least flexible for geriatrics Least flexible for ID CGH	Most flexible for geriatrics Most flexible for ID Southside	Less flexible than 1 & 2 for geriatrics Moder-ately flexible for ID Adults: CGH Children: Gordon's	As 4 for geriatrics and ID Southside]

Note: We have added to the original table by indicating, in square brackets, the scores from Table 7.4, the location of ID provision, and the relevant anomalies.
Source: Adapted from Akehurst 1986: 42–5.

objective is given as 1. Therefore the weighted score (the figure in parentheses) should be 13 (13 × 1). But the figure in Table 7.4 is 22.

Anomaly 2 concerns the score given to Option 6 for 'ease of staffing'. The descriptive gloss for the score given in Table 7.5 simply reads 'As [option] 2'. But while the given score for Option 2 is 7, for Option 6 it is only 1.

Anomaly 3 is concerned with the score for 'flexibility' achieved by Option 1. In Table 7.5 the verbal rating for infectious diseases provision given to Option 1 reads 'most flexible for ID [infectious diseases]'. The description of the criteria used for rating reads, 'For ID, Southside is the most flexible and CGH [Crompton General] the least'. But under Option 1, facilities for infectious diseases would be provided at Crompton General rather then Southside (Akehurst 1986: 25). It follows that the appropriate rating for Option 1 is '*least* flexible for ID'.

Anomaly 4 concerns the score achieved by Option 2 for the 'services to the elderly' objective. Table 7.4 gives this score as 6 and the weighting for this objective as 25. The weighted score should therefore be 150 (6 × 25). But the number we are given is 175.

Anomalies 2 and 3 are, perhaps, harder to recognize as such than are 1 and 4. The latter pair immediately can be seen and explained as 'numerical errors'. The oddity of anomaly 2, however, consists of a disjunction between the verbal information presented in Table 7.5 and the numerical scoring in Table 7.4, while the problem of anomaly 3 is that of a mismatch between three conflicting pieces of verbal information – the rating, the criterial description and the correct ID location.

Of all four, the most straightforward is anomaly 1, which concerns the 'A and E' score assigned to Option 6. The weighted score of 22 given in Table 7.4 can be explained as a 'straightforward error' or 'typo' (note the correct figure of 22 for 'acute services') and can be resolved by adjusting the figure to its correct value of 13 (the weight of 13 multiplied by the score of 1). The consequence of this resolution is, of course, to reduce the total score for Option 6 from 322 to 313. The significance of this result, however, is not great: as Option 6 was said to be rejected because of its 'unacceptably low benefit score' (ibid.: 5) then a further reduction in its benefit score would only serve to strengthen this rationale.

Anomaly 2, which concerns the 'ease of staffing' score for Option 6, is more complicated. The problem is the apparent lack of fit between the words 'As [option] 2' in Table 7.5 and the numbers '1 (9)' as given in Table 7.4. Although this can be explained as *some* kind of error, just what kind is unclear. This difficulty of explanation leads to an equivalent difficulty of resolution. One way is to privilege the words of Table 7.5 over the numbers of Table 7.4. In other words, we can read 'As 2' literally and resolve the problem by replacing the given score of '1 (9)' with the score for Option 2, that is '7 (63)'. The consequence of so doing is that the total score for Option 6 is increased by 54 points to 367 points.[5] As this result makes Option 6's benefit score 45 points *higher* than the original total, one can ask whether this higher score still qualifies as 'unacceptably low'. This is a significant question because, if the new total was judged to be acceptable, Option 6 would become, given its cheapness, the preferred option. Luckily, the increase in score seems too small relative to the scores of the other options to warrant any such reassessment.[6]

We come now to the most significant pair of anomalies which taken together would seem to force a re-evaluation of the outcome of the appraisal. Anomaly 3, concerning the flexibility of Option 1's ID provision, can be explained as the result of a simple error: the word 'most' in the description in Table 7.5 is a mistake; the correct term is 'least'. Once this mistake has been made the error is carried over into the high score of 8 given to Option 1 for flexibility. On the assumption that the two flexibility issues – geriatrics and ID – carry equal weight, we can arrive at a corrected score of 5 for Option 1 as follows:

Most + most (options 4 and 6) = 9. Therefore 'most' = 4.5
Moderate + most (option 2) = 8. Therefore 'moderate' = 3.5
Least + least (option 3) = 3. Therefore 'least' = 1.5
Therefore:
moderate + least (option 1) = 3.5 + 1.5 = 5.

Thus the new weighted score to be given to Option 1 for flexibility is 20 (5 × 4), a reduction of 12 from the original, which gives an adjusted total of 690 points for Option 1. The upshot of this resolution of anomaly 3 is that the difference in the benefit scores of Options 1 (690) and 2 (707) is now 17 points. This degree of difference would, presumably, be much harder to characterize as 'slight' than the original, but seemingly mistaken, difference of 5 points. It appears therefore that Option 2 is beginning to emerge as a clear winner instead of Option 1. However, we have yet to consider the last of the major anomalies.

Anomaly 4, which concerns services to the elderly under Option 2, is the most interesting because it apparently can be resolved in either of two opposed yet equally plausible ways. The anomaly seems to be the result of a simple numerical error: the weight of 25 multiplied by the score of 6 does not equal the given weighted score of 175. But because 175 is a multiple of 25, the anomaly can be resolved by either A, changing the score to 7; or B, changing the weighted score to 150. It can readily be seen that the choice between A and B is highly significant. If we choose to change the score (resolution A) then both the weighted score of 175 and the total benefit score for Option 2 of 707 points remain the same. Taking into account the reduction in the total for Option 1 entailed in the resolution of anomaly 3 as discussed above, this resolution would make the choice of Option 1 over Option 2 even harder to warrant than our earlier analysis, based on the original totals, shows it to be. If, on the other hand, we choose to alter the weighted score (resolution B), then

Table 7.6 Selections from the benefit score matrix: clinicians' course version

Objectives	*Options*			
	Weight	*1*	2	3
Services to the elderly	25	9 (225)	6 (150)	8 (200)
[All other objectives and scores identical to those in Table 7.4]				
Total weighted score (out of 1000)		727	682	663

the total benefit score for Option 2 is reduced by 25 points to 682. This would have the effect of making Option 1 (following the rejection of Option 6) automatically selectable even if we take into account the reduction in its total score produced by resolving anomaly 3: Option 1 would then be both the cheapest – by £109,000 total AEC from Option 2 – and the most beneficial, by 2 points from Option 3.

Unfortunately, there is absolutely nothing elsewhere in *Planning Hospital Services* to guide us in this choice. The determined reader has to go beyond the text at this point – or give up. After finding no assistance in the guideline literature, or in the other published option appraisals, we went to the author of PHS for help.

At a seminar for senior clinicians, at which one of us (Ashmore) was present, recording the events on videotape, the author presented a version of Table 7.4 to illustrate the procedure for weighting, scoring and aggregating benefits.[7] He showed only that part of the table representing Options 1, 2 and 3. From viewing the videotape it was clear that the author had effectively 'resolved the anomaly' by 'correcting' the weighted score (see Table 7.6). In other words, the figures for Option 2's services to the elderly read: 6(150).

However, as our above use of scare quotes indicates, we feel it is unlikely that this 'correction' of the published weighted score can be usefully characterized as a 'resolution of an anomaly', chiefly because the change to the services to the elderly figures for Option 2 was not the only alteration: the corresponding figures for Options 1 and 3 were also changed. They read 9(225) for Option 1 and 8(200) for Option 3. The three new totals were accordingly as follows – Option 1: 727; Option 2: 682; and Option 3: 663. With these figures, of course, there could be no discussion about which option should be selected. Assuming no change in the cost figures, Option 1 looks clearly superior. Nevertheless, in order to accept its superiority, one must treat the new figures as entirely trustworthy. But, of course, these could well have been ungrounded adjustments made for the sake of clarity in a teaching context.

Accordingly, our next step was to ask the author directly if he could help us to resolve anomaly 4. After examining the text he said that he would be much more confident in the weighted score of 175 than in the score of 6.[8] As we have seen above, by leaving Option 2's total score unchanged, this decision, in conjunction with the reduced total for Option 1 attendant on resolving anomaly 3, once again makes the original selection of the latter option in PHS extremely difficult to justify. It seems that the more closely and carefully we examine the practical recommendations generated by this exemplary appraisal, the less clear, the less convincing and the less rational does it become.

A positive conclusion

So far we have attempted to disrupt the given basis for the choice of Option 1 by challenging the author's quantitative rhetoric, by showing how the use of a different set of costs would affect the outcome and by demonstrating the vulnerability of the benefit scores to changes resulting from close attention to anomalies. In this section we make some positive suggestions about the likely grounds of choice. In particular, we document our earlier suggestion that the choice hinged on a general preference, other things being sufficiently equal, for low cost over high benefit. We further suggest that this abstract preference was given weight by the selective, and political, attention to one particular cost criterion.

We have three points to make about the preference for low cost over high benefit. The first concerns the general form of the question to be asked by decision-makers when confronted with a choice of the kind we are examining. If no option is clearly superior, it is typically suggested in the guideline literature that the choice should be dependent on the answer to the following kind of question: is the higher benefit worth the higher cost? (Henderson 1984: 25). This question is fleshed out in Akehurst's recent review of the appraisal process (Akehurst 1987). In the absence of a superior option, the choice 'depends on the extra points "bought" for the extra money and the alternative uses of the extra money. . . . The crucial question is what would the extra [money] buy for patients if spent in some other way. A judgement has to be made about which set of benefits that can be bought is the more worthwhile' (ibid.: 16–17). In other words, judgements about the opportunity cost of the extra money have to be made. However, one may ask how these additional judgements are to be made. After all, an option appraisal is usually recommended as the best way of deciding 'which set of benefits . . . is the more worthwhile'. If a second appraisal is required to settle the issue of the first appraisal, and this second appraisal is also inconclusive, as is more than likely, then it would seem that a regress of appraisals is set in train that would only cease when one of them happened to throw up a clearly superior option.[9]

Of course, an infinite regress of option appraisals is not what is recommended. Instead, some other unspecified way of making the required judgements is called for. Indeed, it is precisely at this point – the point at which adjudication between two or more non-superior options is necessary – that a space is opened for the exercise of the kind of managerial judgement required to sustain the rhetoric of option appraisal as a decision-aiding tool as opposed to a decision-making machine. In the unusual case of an appraisal which 'works', in that it produces a superior option, there is no opportunity for the exercise of such judgement. Thus, while it is important for the credibility of the 'weak rhetoric' of decision-aiding that appraisals should be, and usually are, 'unsuccessful', the necessity in such cases for employing some other way of making the final choice casts doubt on the credibility of the 'strong rhetoric' which emphasizes the superiority of the more rational, more explicit and more systematic process of option appraisal as compared to these alternative modes of choice.

However, it could be argued that the 'alternative modes of choice' employed at this stage will not really be very different, in their spirit at least, from those used in the appraisal, given the type of question which decision-makers are recommended to ask themselves in those cases when an appraisal fails to produce a winner. The question, 'Is the higher benefit worth the higher cost?' is strictly limited in its applicability to options with the higher-benefit/higher-cost characteristic. In the case we are examining, as represented in the figures of Table 7.1, it could be asked of Option 2 but not of Option 1. The recommended re-examination, then, is one-sided: an equivalent reassessment of the alternative option – the one with lower benefit and lower cost – is *not* suggested. In practice, this asymmetry seems likely to result, on at least some occasions, in *deciding against* the option which has been subject to question. That which is questioned is clearly more vulnerable to revision than that which is not. Moreover, that which is not questioned may seem by that very fact to be superior to that which is, literally, questionable.

This asymmetric situation could, of course, be remedied precisely by asking an equivalent question of the option with the lower-benefit/lower-cost characteristic. As we have found no guidelines for formulating such a question, we have attempted the task ourselves. At first we simply substituted the term 'lower' for the term 'higher' in the original question, thus: is the lower benefit worth the lower cost? We soon realized that this formulation was unsatisfactory. Because a 'lower benefit' is a cost and a 'lower cost' is a benefit – and because cost–benefit thinking always assesses the benefit by reference to the cost and never the other way round – our preferred formulation of the alternative question is this: is the (benefit of the) lower cost worth the (cost of the) lower benefit? It would be interesting to speculate about the outcome of the appraisal had this question been asked of Option 1.

A rather more specific point concerns the way in which the 'Do Nothing' option is treated. As we have seen, the summary states that this option 'has been rejected because of its unacceptably low benefit score' (Akehurst 1986: 5). This brief statement is expanded to almost an entire page in the 'Overall Comparison of Options' section (ibid.: 47–9). The expansion includes a detailed examination of the ways in which 'doing nothing' except reducing beds to target requirements would, rather unsurprisingly, fail to achieve the four major service improvements listed as objectives B–E above (ibid.: 48). The relevant question is why, *given* this option's 'unacceptably low benefit score', any further discussion – or indeed, any discussion at all – was necessary. The answer would appear to be simply because Option 6 was also the cheapest. Rejecting the least costly option clearly requires more extensive justification than does rejecting the option which gives the greatest benefit.

Third, the overt political context of the appraisal – that of a rationalization of services – makes the requirement to reduce costs the paramount consideration. Moreover, it leads to the role of the appraisal as a *political* tool being made explicit. For example, in the case of acute services, it is stated that:

> The City Strategy, Regional Strategy and Regional Review all require a large reduction in the number of acute beds in the District. . . . Achieving this reduction in the face of opposition from staff and clinicians is likely to prove a very difficult task indeed, unless some offer of improvement can be made in the quality of stock, in order to compensate for the loss of quantity.
> (ibid.: 12)

Comments such as this (see also ibid.: 4 and 51) strongly suggest that the initial framework of the appraisal made considerations of reduced cost the priority and that any benefits that may have been forthcoming were essentially subordinate to that primary concern.

Finally, we would like to suggest that there is one particular cost criterion which, although it is never applied explicitly to Option 2, could have been used to eliminate this option from further consideration. The criterion is that of 'efficiency' (see Table 7.2, row D), which is described as follows in the 'Comment on Overall Priority':

> In Regional terms the highest priority category given to schemes is those in which significant sums of revenue will be released by gains to be made in efficiency. The strategy quantifies this as applying to

> savings in excess of £100,000 p.a., and in the case of [Option 1] the efficiency savings are £306,000 p.a. putting the scheme at the head of this category.[10]
>
> (ibid.: 17)

Looking at Table 7.2, we can see that the efficiency savings for Option 2 are given as £98,000; that is, £2,000 *less* than the figure required to put this option into the 'highest priority category'. If this was the case, we have here an implicit cost criterion which would effectively discriminate against Option 2, but which is not even mentioned in the context of the final choice.

These various indicators of the asymmetry between cost and benefit suggest that here, as in other option appraisals, those involved are able to produce a firm recommendation, not by applying a set of explicit, neutral procedures, but by drawing upon a range of implicit and socially located background assumptions.

Is *Planning Hospital Services* a poor appraisal?

In this section we wish to make it clear that we have not been engaged in this chapter in unmasking technical inadequacy. Nevertheless, we feel it important to address the impression, gained from responses to earlier presentations of this analysis, that this is precisely what we have been doing. The fact that we have been able to deconstruct some features of PHS does not imply that the text was, in its technical aspects, especially 'ripe' for such treatment. *Any* analytical artefact is in principle subject to deconstruction – as rival experimentalists in the natural sciences know well. Indeed, what we have been doing is nothing more than what participants themselves do in the course of a scientific controversy. A close inspection of experimental or technical procedures will soon start to reveal difficulties and ambiguities (Pinch 1986; Collins 1985). The inevitable effect of drawing attention to the judgements and implicit practices which underlie the surface rationality of PHS is to make this example of an option appraisal seem technically inadequate. We realize, moreover, that participants themselves may wish to defend the general procedures of option appraisal by reading our text as a technical evaluation and by attributing any supposed defects to the peculiarities of this particular example.

However, we have to admit that there is one particular sense in which PHS is indeed more deconstructable than other published option appraisals. We refer to its textual representation of a decision. This aspect of the text, as we mentioned above, makes it a particularly apposite focus for an analysis of the relation between appraisals and decisions. However, the existence of the decision alongside the appraisal allowed us to treat the 'gap' between these two components of PHS in an ironic fashion. This entailed our showing how the appraisal reported in PHS failed to live up to the strong-programme rhetoric of clear, rational calculation which presents option appraisal as a superior and apolitical decision-making procedure. But in ironicizing this 'failure', we ourselves failed to do justice to participants' weak-programme rhetoric in which option appraisal is depicted as a decision-aiding tool which necessarily has to operate in a political environment. Moreover, and paradoxically, the 'failure' of our efforts on behalf of the lay reader to extract an unalloyed logic of appraisal from PHS can be seen as 'successfully' revealing the uncertainty, equivocation and compromise which, according to the weak programme, are inescapable in the real world of practical action.

A brief lesson

If we wish to have a system of planning and decision-making in which the kinds of tensions we have discussed in this chapter – between appraisal and politics, decision-making and decision-aiding, and technical adequacy and practical utility – are dissolved, we can choose to (a) dispense with option appraisal and all the other manifestations of applied economic rationality dealt with in this book and revert to 'the mixture as before', or (b) impose the rigours of economic analysis wholesale on the system. If, on the other hand, and after due consideration, we reach the conclusion, for example, that (a) is undesirable and (b) practically impossible, then we must realize that this entails the cost, if it is a cost, of recognizing and taking account of the ways in which the tensions and dualities that have been our topic throughout this book will continue to operate to frustrate both the over-rational expectations of some proponents of applied social science as well as the more apocalyptic fears of its opponents. It is to considerations such as these that we turn our attention in the next and final chapter.

Notes

1. This quotation is from a talk by R. Akehurst on 'Option Appraisal' given at the course for clinicians held at Bowness-on-Windermere in March 1986. See Chapter 6, note 1, for details.
2. Guidance material issued by the government include DHSS 1981b, 1987a; Burchell and Gilbert 1982; Treasury 1984. Similar material published by health economists include Akehurst and Buxton 1985; Henderson 1984; Henderson and Mooney 1984.

3. Reviews of current practice include DHSS 1987b; Ludbrook and Mooney 1984; Mooney and Henderson 1984; Culyer 1985b; Akehurst 1987; Alban 1982; Ludbrook 1984.
4. The objective of improving out-patient services was the subject of a separate 'sub-option appraisal' and does not figure in Akehurst's paper or our analysis.
5. This is a cumulative total; that is, it takes into account the previous result for anomaly 1.
6. Alternative resolutions of anomaly 2 are more difficult. For instance, privileging the score of 1 over the 'As 2' (the reverse of the present procedure) warrants some statement to the effect that 'doing nothing' will entail massive difficulties with staffing. From the information available in PHS, however, it is difficult to construct a statement, equivalent to those given for the other options, to this effect. Another possible resolution involves discounting both 'As 2' and the score on the grounds that the error involved the mistaken substitution of 'As 2' for 'As 4'; Option 4 being similar to Option 6 in that both are 'four-site solutions' (Akehurst 1983: 36, 38). This resolution would therefore give Option 6 the same score as Option 4, that is, '4(36)'.
7. The seminar (see Ch. 6, note 1) took place in March 1986. *Planning Hospital Services* was published in January 1986.
8. This is a paraphrase from notes taken later.
9. Health economists recognize, however, that this kind of result is rare (Akehurst 1987: 16; Akehurst and Buxton 1985: 6). All six of the published option appraisals we have cited produced inconclusive results. This situation, of course, merely testifies to the general validity of such maxims of vulgar economics as 'you get what you pay for'.
10. The statement that the efficiency savings accruing to Option 1 puts the scheme 'at the head of this category' constitutes yet another anomaly. From Table 7.2, row D, it can be seen that Option 3, with an efficiency saving of £356,000 p.a., is £50,000 p.a. more efficient than Option 1.

8 Summaries, conclusions and readings

In the course of this study, we have tried to enter into the culture of the community of British health economists. One of our central aims has been to try to understand health economists' professional life from the inside. Thus in this book we have sought to convey a rich sense of their tasks, as they see them, their methods, their conceptions of the social world, their successes and their failures. In the preceding chapters we have tried to give ample expression to the many voices of health economists on a range of general and specific issues by quoting at length from recorded interviews, from published papers and unpublished reports, from videotapes of their varied activities, from articles in the press, and from radio and television programmes.

At the same time, we have also tried to step back and to view health economics from the outside. We must stress, however, that looking at health economists 'from the outside' is not the same as 'providing a definitive account' of their social practices. We mean, rather, that we have tried to use our understanding of the culture of health economics to identify features and to reveal relationships which are characteristic of that culture as we see it, but which are not recognized, or not explicitly formulated, or perhaps even denied, in the discourse of health economists themselves. In other words, in this study, we have attempted to do justice to participants' own views of their activities, but also to depict these activities as they appear from our alternative position in the world of social science.

Although our study is unusual in that both the investigators and the subjects are social scientists, its concerns and implications have a much wider relevance. For we have been dealing with the application of social science to a field of action which involves all members of society at critical junctures of their lives. Furthermore, it seems that social scientists often claim to speak about such matters on behalf of the community at large. It seemed to us essential, therefore, to allow into our text at least some non-social scientists so that they could express their own views and make clear that the voice of the social scientist, whether economist or sociologist, operates from a perspective which differs significantly from that of 'ordinary people'.

Broadly speaking, then, three different perspectives on health economics and its practical consequences have been built into the analysis above; namely, that of the sociologist, that of the health economist, and that of the layperson. But this threefold division should not be taken to imply that each of these perspectives is unified and internally coherent. For example, our approach to sociological research, with its emphasis on multiple voices and on the diversity of possible interpretations, is quite alien to some members of our own discipline. In their hands, the sociological study of health economics would bear little resemblance to the present text. Similarly, not only are there different versions of health economics available among its practitioners, but, as we have stressed, each participant is able to formulate his or her own practice and the nature of health economics differently in varying circumstances. Finally, to refer to 'the layperson's' perspective on health economics is merely a way of drawing attention to the existence of a great range of socially located responses of which we gave a hint in Chapters 4 and 5 but which lay largely outside the restricted scope of our study.

In previous chapters we have tried to weave these discrepant multidimensional voices into our representation of health economics. Undoubtedly our own analytical voice has been dominant and has obscured those of the health economists and, even more, the voices of other interested parties. In a text of this kind, it is impossible to avoid exaggerating the importance of one's own limited perspective. But the situation would be made even worse if, in this final chapter, we claimed the exclusive right to draw things together and to impose our own, uncontested view of the social practice of health economics. Consequently, we provide three different 'readings' of the book from the perspectives of an economist, a sociologist and a layperson. Before we do so, however, we would like to present our own brief summary of the study together with our assessment of the implications that it holds for the practice of applied social science.

Summaries and conclusions (with imaginary interruptions)

In this book we have portrayed health economists, as they attempt to apply their specialist knowledge in the practical domain of health care, as actors who are forced to confront the series of dilemmas, paradoxes and tensions we have identified and who have therefore developed the threefold strategy described in Chapter 1. In Chapter 2 we specified how the educative strategy depends for its success on its practitioners being able to negotiate the 'dual programme of health economics'. If their audience of health care professionals are to be persuaded of the benefits of health economics, health economists have to formulate the argument that current health care practices are deficient, and that only the discipline of economics can greatly improve things, without thereby alienating those whom they criticize. Mooney and Drummond resolved this dilemma of application by their skilful intermingling of the strong and the weak programmes.

MD: So skilful, in fact, that we ourselves who actually wrote the series of articles which you analyse at such great length were totally unaware that we were 'intermingling the strong and weak programmes'. We hope it is not too late to point out that while you use the terms 'strong' and 'weak' frequently, you have nowhere provided a definitive account of the features of your so-called 'dual programme'.

The main features of the dual programme can be represented as a series of dichotomies as in Table 8.1.

MD: That's made things a lot clearer. Now we can all see what you're driving at. And we're happy to accept your generous assessment of our contribution to the process of educating health care professionals. It is

Table 8.1 The dual programme of health economics

Strong programme	*Weak programme*
Radical wholesale change of current practices	Small-scale gradual change necessitated by accommodation to current practices
Economic thought needed by everyone	Economics and economists as useful technical aids
Systematic research	Quick and dirty research
Testing and experimentation	Learning from experience
Clear-cut successes and failures which can be independently evaluated	Failure and success hard to judge – evaluation inseparable from implementation
One rational way of speaking and acting (the model of the calculative rational actor)	Multiple ways of speaking and acting each with their own rationality
Politics as an unfortunate distortion of rational action	Politics as a necessary form of mediation, negotiation and persuasion between groups with different rational expectations

noticeable, however, that you haven't made a habit of commending the work of health economists. Did you get increasingly disenchanted, or what?

That's an interesting question. The answer is that we have become more and more aware of the ambiguities of our task and especially of the role of evaluation within it. As symmetrical analysts in the sociology of scientific knowledge tradition (see Bloor 1976; Collins 1985; Knorr-Cetina and Mulkay 1983; Ashmore 1989) we refuse, on principle, to evaluate the epistemological status of the knowledge claims we analyse. However, as applied sociologists of expertise we find that to avoid all evaluation of health economics is as unsatisfactory as it is impossible.

MD: So despite the rhetoric, you just think that we practise bad science?

Certainly not! Though, as Chapter 6 shows, it took some of us some considerable time to stop comparing health economics with physics. No, it's not the epistemological status of applied economics in any abstract sense that concerns us but rather the specific moral and political implications of its underlying assumptions. This leads us to be critical of the culture of economic evaluation in almost all spheres and not least in health. But simply to get involved in writing an academic critique cum political tract, and thus damning the lot of you – no offence intended – would be to play the game you health economists play. For example, we would then become involved in offering our own solutions for the problems of health care provision, which is something that is not our task as analysts of health economics. Furthermore, if we were to list the 'ills of health economics' in precisely the same way that you specify those of the NHS, it would be difficult for us to create any radically new approach to applied social science.

MD: We'll look forward to seeing you do that. In the meantime, we'll have to get back to our important work in health economics; though we're most grateful for this unusual opportunity to intervene.

Speaking of which, in Chapter 3 we dealt with the strategy of direct intervention. First, we attended to the ways in which the economists' model of the individual rational actor is used as the basis for attributing various degrees of irrationality to the NHS as a whole. We then examined how health economists fared in their attempts to raise the level of rationality in the system either by entering the NHS and working on the inside or by offering their skills as external researchers or consultants. We found that their efforts were constantly hampered by their dependence on the very system they wished to change. Moreover, their identity as *economists* – bearers of both a special 'bag of tools' and a distinctive 'way of thinking' – was continually threatened by the practical need to accommodate to the immediate requirements of their bureaucratic role or their customers' research protocol. In short, they faced the 'dilemma of the quick and dirty': in order to be able to exercise their economic expertise at all they had to compromise the particular character and larger aims of that expertise.

8.1

Aggrieved, unquoted and uncategorizable health economist: I want to have my say here having been unselected for comment in Chapter 3. Although I have many interesting things to say about we health economists' attempts at 'direct intervention in the NHS' as you somewhat grandiosely put it, I think it would be more useful at this juncture to discuss methodology. You sociologists are supposed to be interested in the topic, especially as it is *your* methodology I wish to talk about (see my colleague Tony Culyer's [1985c] piece). Whether Chapter 3's 'quote and commentary' form of presentation within which I am trapped allows for it or not, I would like to start by asking you a direct question. How did you select the quotes you used and what warrant have you for claiming they are 'exemplary'?

This participant complains that s/he was not called upon to give his or her views in a previous chapter and on these grounds claims the right to speak here. S/he then changes the topic of discussion to 'our methodology' and insists that because we are sociologists we are bound to be fascinated with this topic. After claiming to be 'trapped' in an unsuitable 'form of presentation', s/he offers to begin the discussion with 'a direct question'. However, it is noticeable that s/he proceeds to ask *two* questions, not one. The participant continues, as we see in the next passage, by maintaining that the 'question(s)' s/he has asked have not received a satisfactory answer.

8.2

. . . haven't answered my question – alright, questions – at all. This form of presentation, as I suspected, does not seem to allow for dialogue, let alone 'collaborative analysis' (see your earlier paper claiming that you engage in such analysis [Ashmore *et al.* 1988] which was even 'co-authored' by myself and colleagues [members of the Health Economists' Study Group]). But, as an experienced applied social scientist used to talking with recalcitrant clinicians who fail to understand the simplest point, I will try again. Let me put it this way. You selected the quotes you used in Chapter 3 because they allowed you to tell a story of problems. No doubt in *some* sense they were indeed 'exemplary': there *are* a lot of problems as I know very well. But what I doubt is that your corpus of transcripts did not contain sufficient, and sufficiently exemplary, material with which, had you chosen to use it, you could have told a different story: perhaps, even, a story of triumphal success. Clearly, this did not suit your purpose. It seems to me, therefore, that the story you told is your story, not ours. You did not so much 'discover' it as 'invent' it. And your talk at the beginning of the chapter of 'data', of 'illustration' and 'documentation' is, therefore, a misrepresentation of your practice. You would no doubt say in response, if you could, that I am largely correct in this analysis, but that you did not intend to misrepresent your practice which is indeed 'constructive' (your preferred metaphor). Indeed, you could continue, it is specified in Chapter 1 that a partial story is all that is available to any teller be s/he health economist or sociologist. And in any case, as you might wish to point out, more than one story is told in the book (though admittedly, they all have a similar theme) and more than one textual form is used to tell them; and, if plays, dialogues and detailed technical deconstructions can be used, why not this form of interview analysis with its mildly empiricist, yet surely harmless, connotations. And finally, you may well conclude, why should an *economist* object to such a form?

As we tried to do throughout Chapter 3, we have allowed this participant to speak for him or herself. In any case, there is little we can usefully add to such a perspicuous analysis. Let us therefore return to our summary.

Our presentation of the strategy of public debate in Chapter 4 showed once again how the context in which health economists have to operate – in this case, the mass media – crucially affects the outcome. In this forum, the resort to the dual rhetoric is seldom an option. Because the media tends to simplify technical discourse and to polarize technical argument, only the strongest messages are noticed, which are then duly taken to task for their outrageousness. The economists' arguments for increased rationality in health care provision, seem, in this setting, to be as irrational as those of their opponents. What we might call the 'paradox of public presentation' means that continued efforts to get the message across entail massively increased risks that the message will be distorted beyond recognition and thus will *not* get across.

Our reporters comment: This calumny on the press cannot be allowed to pass uncontested. Most of us in our profession scrupulously attempt to report the events of the world with accuracy and sensitivity. We also have a duty to represent all shades of opinion and to maintain, as far as we are able, a balanced approach. We must balance not only opposing views, but opposing roles. We must inform and yet entertain. We must report and at the same time we must comment. We have to satisfy our employers, our advertisers and our customers. We have to sell newspapers or television programmes and yet we must endeavour to maintain the integrity of the third estate, that bulwark against unfreedom. Ours is not an easy job.

This is not to say that we necessarily would want to dispute the thrust of your analysis. For amateurs you did quite well. The health economists do not, we think, emerge with their rationality intact. But then, who does?

In Chapters 5, 6 and 7 we have shown how these paradoxes, tensions and dilemmas are constitutive, not just of the strategies health economists have used in order to open up a space for the effective application of their knowledge and skills, but of some of the specific forms which this application takes. In Chapter 5, for example, we demonstrated how the QALY . . .

Not to my satisfaction, you didn't. It seems to me that you failed to 'demonstrate' anything in Chapter 5. In fact you made a point of refusing to do so. You insisted that your discussion of the QALY was simply that: a discussion.

Yes, indeed. And that's one of the points we were about to reiterate. You see, what we have written so far in this concluding chapter is again only a version of . . .

'Only a version'! What a debilitating doctrine that is!

We're sorry you feel like that about it. But, of course, the 'doctrine' as you call it is really much more complex and interesting than your dismissive summary would suggest. What we are saying is . . .

. . . only a version.

. . . that the social world is itself a paradoxical and multivocal phenomenon . . .

. . . which is a view which neither the economists nor myself ('the questioning voice of the potential recipient') hold because in order to do any work in the world we have to believe that it is, for all practical purposes, understandable and manipulable in the terms of a unitary discourse such as, for example, economics.

. . . constituted and deconstituted by a complex and constantly changing concatenation of voices and versions of which this is just one . . .

I knew you were going to say that.

. . . or rather several. Therefore, in order to be true to this version of the character of the social world, we are obliged to attempt multivocal analysis, to recover some of the variation in the accounts we are given, to use a variety of textual forms, and to attend to issues of reflexivity.

But you haven't been listening, as usual. You would be much more convincing if you dealt with the points I raise rather than just giving us the benefit of your own unalloyed strong programme. A bit more thought and rather fewer slogans would help. So how about a response to the need for unitary discourse in the realm of practical affairs?

Certainly. Throughout the book we have tried to suggest that the comparative lack of progress of applied health economics – compared, that is, to our initial estimate of its favourable prospects – can be explained by health economists' lack of attention to the implications of their own weak programme. In practice, as we have seen, the economists' clear desire to impose their own unitary discourse tends to be undermined, and that discourse itself subverted, by that other discourse with which they come into contact at every turn and which it is their aim, in strong-programme terms, to change. This is the discourse of day-to-day practice, the discourse of professional power, the discourse of politics; in short, to economists it is the discourse of irrationality. Yet the only way that they can hope to get the bearers of this other discourse to think and act like economists, which is essential for the success of applied economics, is to accommodate to the practical exigencies of the everyday world. They must persuade because they cannot force. They must sell their products to a sophisticated market which is quite capable of rejecting them out of hand. They must depict their products as helpful, unthreatening or, best of all, necessary. These modes of accommodation we have called the weak programme. Many health economists seem to treat the need to engage in weak programme discourse as an unpleasant and, it is hoped, temporary charade which can be abandoned once it has achieved its purpose – such Machiavellian political metaphors as the iron fist in the velvet glove or the poisoned chalice come to mind. Others are changed, and in differing ways chastened, by the experience. Some of these – especially insiders – embrace the 'realism' of the weak programme wholeheartedly and abandon the strong programme of health economics altogether, dismissing it as utopian, unrealistic and, perhaps, as fundamentally misguided. A different reaction, which we have observed most frequently among outsiders, entails a subtle reformulation of the aims of the strong programme. The 'tools' of economic analysis become the means of producing social consensus rather than self-contained technical results; though it is assumed that the consensus thus produced is founded on a common recognition of the adequacy and relevance of the economic way of thinking.

Thus, we can only respond to your point about the necessity for unitary discourse by disagreeing with it. Neither the strong nor the weak programme of health economics is able to survive independently of the other. The practical application of health economics and, we suggest, social science more generally, requires the artful handling of a variety of discourses. The practical social scientist has to be adept at translation, at semantic transformation, at rhetoric; she must be able to acknowledge the full variety of rational action in her chosen domain; she must come to terms with the paradoxes, the dilemmas and the tensions of social life; and she must recognize the essential similarity between her own ways of proceeding and those of the other actors with whom she is concerned.

I see. You seem to be saying something like this, and I paraphrase: 'practical social scientists are deemed to be acting fully rationally and are regarded as capable of achieving their own values most effectively, only in so far as they come to think and act like sociologists'.

Yes, that seems to put it rather well. That, indeed, is our weak programme for an applied sociology of expertise.

Did you say 'weak programme'?

That's right.

I could have sworn it was your strong version. After all, it directly parallels that of the health economists.

Oh no. However strong it looks, that's our weak programme because it is a version that has been formulated in a way which accommodates to the expectation that social science will adopt a unitary form of discourse. To accept and to put forward just one version of events, no matter how agreeable that version may be, is to deny the fundamental insight of (our version of) our discipline, namely that the social world is multiple and paradoxical. Thus, the conclusion to this study which best represents the strong programme of the sociology of expertise is multiple.

For now, however, let us continue our unitary weak-programme summary. In Chapter 5, with the help of our interlocutor, we deconstructed . . .

I beg your pardon?

. . we analysed the assumptions underlying the QALY measure. In particular, we drew attention to the assumptions of aggregate representation, correspondence to reality, stability of preferences and neutrality of quantification. All of these, though highly contestable, seem essential if the meaning ascribed to the QALY by those concerned with its production and use is to be maintained. For instance, the assumption that aggregate data on preferences correctly represent the individual evaluations from which they originate is shown . . .

Careful.

. . . is claimed to be an artefact of the procedures used to collect the data. No single evaluation need coincide with the aggregate representations and . . .

Look, I've said this before but I see it needs saying again. What is your alternative? If you dispense with such measurements how can any applied social science hope to have an effect?

If we social scientists carry on using measurements like these in the face of what are, at least in the sociological community, very well-recognized deficiencies (see, for example, Cicourel 1964), we run the considerable risk of Mrs Jones greeting the latest deluge of figures with a robust 'So what?' (Williams 1987: 566). And surely none of us can afford to greet *that* prospect with an equivalent retort.

But to move on. The social technology of clinical budgeting was our topic in Chapter 6. In this play we attempted to show how every aspect of clinical budgeting – its definition, its purpose, its scientific status, its evaluation and even our own analysis – were subject to systematic variation. Once more using the metaphor of the strong and the weak, we were able to distinguish two basic rhetorics . . .

Researcher Four: Only two again! We would have thought that with your emphasis on the multiple character of the social world you could have managed more than that. Still, you're not the only ones. Dualisms and dichotomies are a favourite device of authors writing in the sociology of scientific knowledge. Consider, for example, the fertility of the constitutive/contingent (Collins and Pinch 1979), the contingent/empiricist (Gilbert and Mulkay 1984) and the Janus-faced device used by Latour (1987).

You're right, such dualities *are* surprisingly fruitful. However, we don't entirely limit ourselves to the strong/weak couple or indeed to dichotomies at all. We deal, you will recall, with health economists' threefold strategy as well as their use of three-part lists. We examine three of their techniques, the book ends with three different 'readings' and, of course, we are a trio of authors.

Researcher Four: Oh, very impressive!

Be that as it may, at the end of Chapter 6, we gave ourselves the task (or rather our three fictional researchers did) of coming to some conclusion about the kind of research practice that we have been engaged in. It may seem strange to some of you that this was not a settled question, especially at such an advanced stage of the book. It may seem even stranger to suggest that the question is not really ours to answer. Whether we are doing 'real science, or "quick and dirty" policy research, or sensitive participant-centred research' is really for you, The Reader, to decide. We have our own views, of course, as Researcher One makes clear at the end of the chapter. But as they really have little relevance to your decision, we have decided not to expand upon them here.

Instead, we will conclude our summary. In Chapter 7 we examined the technique of option appraisal. This relatively well-established procedure for making capital expenditure decisions was represented, for the purposes of our analysis, by the exemplary text, *Planning Hospital Services*. An extremely detailed technical deconstruction of this text enabled us to show that neither the improved rationality of decision-making said to be brought about by option appraisal, nor the claimed rationality of the procedure itself, were straightforwardly evident.

Feeling unsure of the adequacy of this summary of Chapter 7, we asked the author of PHS for his opinion. He said (the following is a paraphrase) that in his opinion our appraisal of his text suffered from an overconcentration on irrelevant detail and failed, in consequence, to do justice to the very real contribution that option appraisal in general can make, and indeed has made, to improving the ways in which capital spending decisions are taken in the NHS and that our harping (or possibly 'carping' – this was unclear) on his use of words like 'slightly' and 'considerably' or on the fact that some secretary inadvertently had committed a numerical error or two was neither here nor there and that for the life of him he could not see how our going on and on about such trivia could possibly help to improve the practice of option appraisal one iota, which should have been, he would have thought, our primary concern just as it was his, and yet he was unable, from his reading of our text, to discern this concern beneath the surface of our analysis, which worried him considerably; though he was pleased to be able to say that two can play at the anomalies game and that he would like to present us with a list of some of our grosser technical errors and misinterpretations.

For our part we want to assure our readers that we have duly rechecked the details of Chapter 7 and have corrected the few insignificant infelicities which were so kindly brought to our attention. More importantly, we would like to point out that the chapter's critical conclusion summarized above was modified by our recognition that it was a product of our own reliance upon a particular 'strong' version of the aims and achievements of the procedure we examined. Our alternative conclusion, therefore, was that option appraisal, and by extension, similar analytical techniques, may be considered relatively successful in the terms of its own weak rhetoric, which recognizes the 'uncertainty, equivocation and compromise which are inescapable in the real world of practical action'.

It is this message which, as we mentioned above, serves as our own 'weak programme for applied social science'. The tensions, dilemmas and paradoxes which the health economists face are, and should be, inescapable. Were it not so we would, all of us, be forced to live in a world dominated by the rampant techniques of the triumphant social technologist. Should we then celebrate the inevitable failure of such a programme? Undoubtedly yes; but this does not mean that applied social science is in itself entirely undesirable. A world which was thought so perfect that there was no point in trying to improve it – a Panglossian world – is as profoundly disquieting as its opposite; and perhaps even more so. Efforts at reform and change must, and will, continue. Applied social scientists of all kinds will continue to make a major contribution to these efforts. And as they do so, they will, like the health economists, be faced with the fundamental problem that the very practices they wish to alter will tend to frustrate their efforts.

The point we wish to emphasize is that confronting this 'problem', if it is understood in the way we suggest in this book, is the essential first step towards a better form of practice (if we may be permitted such a blatant evaluation): one that consists of a willingness to work with, rather than against, the actors in the domain of application; one that is collaborative rather than imperious; modest rather than megalomaniac; and wishing to learn rather than itching to instruct.

This brings to an end the authors' concluding summary. In view of the interruptions which occurred in the course of this summary, as well as the possibly confusing diversity of perspectives in some of the prior chapters, we now offer three coherent readings of the text in the hope that they will help you to reach a conclusion, or conclusions, of your own.

Rational affirmation: an economist's reading

This case study by Ashmore, Mulkay and Pinch (AMP) shows just how difficult, but also how necessary, it is to use the intellectual fruits of the advanced social sciences to help solve the practical problems of the everyday social world. It is necessary because human beings are faced with unavoidable problems of scarcity and choice in all areas of social life, including that of health care, and because the most effective answers to these problems can only be established by means of detached, systematic and precise analysis. It is difficult because human behaviour in the aggregate is inefficient and persistently irrational to such an extent that ordinary participants are frequently unable, or unwilling, to implement rational solutions when they are made available.

As an economist, I do not mean to suggest, of course, that people are irrational in the sense of not seeking to maximise their own level of satisfaction or welfare. In fact, we know that most human conduct, particularly in the economic sphere, involves a rational use of means in relation to ends by the individual actors involved. But individuals operate within complex social settings where information about the actions of other parties, and about the consequences of one's own actions, is often lacking; and where the structure of incentives often encourages choices which reduce the level of collective output below that possible with a more efficient distribution of effort. These structurally generated inefficiencies are likely to be particularly evident in cases like the provision of health care services in Britain. For in the British health care system, the end-product is normally provided free for the recipient, whilst its production and delivery depend on the operation of a large, internally divided and cumbersome bureaucracy.

In the preceding chapters, AMP have shown how health economists have begun to use the findings of academic economics to improve the NHS by making it work more efficiently. Health economists have been able to do this because they have command of a set of economic principles and analytical tools which express in scientific form certain basic social realities that are, at best, only partly visible to the untrained layperson. The long-term aim of health economists is to use their expertise to devise accurate measures of costs and benefits (e.g. by means of QALYs, clinical budgeting and option appraisal) which can be employed within the NHS in such a way that, with any given allocation of public resources, the provision of benefit for society at large will be at the highest possible level.

AMP have not hesitated to draw attention to health economists' failures and inadequacies; and quite rightly so. But the most basic problem in this field of applied social science is not of the economists' making; it is, rather, built into the very nature of the situation with which they are faced. For the health economists' guiding aim is to provide rational solutions for an organization which needs their help precisely because it is incapable of acting rationally. In other words, the very process of application, namely, using rational argument to convince irrational people to behave rationally, poses a fundamental challenge to the applied economist. We may call this the paradox of applied rationality. Health economists have not yet solved this paradox. This is because the paradox of applied rationality is not a theoretical problem, to be dealt with by means of elegant abstract analysis, but a recurrent practical difficulty, to be overcome only by means of determined collective effort. Perhaps the biggest failure, therefore, of the British health economists has been that of underestimating the scale and likely duration of their remedial task.

In the chapters above, AMP succeed in conveying just how unreceptive is the British health care system and, indeed, the wider society to the practical changes needed to make the NHS more efficient. They also show us how the health economists have been forced constantly to adjust and to compromise in order to bring about even minor improvements in the delivery of health care. The fundamental reason for this is that few participants in the health care system are able to take the wider view that is automatically adopted by the trained and independent economist. Health care workers are part of a complex, highly differentiated division of labour and, in the case of clinicians, belong to a narrow coterie of medical expertise. Accordingly, their preferences and their choices inevitably reflect their limited perspective and, in many cases, their sectional interest. Of course economists, especially those who work within the bureaucracy, are not entirely free of these limitations. Yet their basic intellectual skills require them to seek, not some narrowly conceived advantage, but the most efficient use of resources for the system as a whole. However, although they constantly strive for this goal, it is not their task as health economists to implement their own recommendations. They depend for this, as AMP clearly demonstrate, upon endorsement from other, more powerful parties within the health care system. As a result, their contributions are always mediated through, and often distorted by, the administrative and political processes of the NHS.

In the first half of this book, the authors describe and document in a fairly straightforward manner the difficulties experienced by health economists both inside and outside the formal system of health care and in the public debate about the future of the NHS. In the later chapters, they provide critical accounts of three of the major techniques used by economists to raise the level of operational rationality within the health care system. It is in these chapters that their analysis is at its weakest. In the first place, they are inclined to adopt here an unnecessarily elaborate and uneconomical style of presentation which may be partly responsible for their persistent failure to adopt the essential distinction between health economists' theoretical solutions to the problems of the NHS and their achievements in practice. This failure prevents AMP from recognizing that, although health economists' practical achievements are as yet somewhat limited, their solutions in principle are not only rational, but are bound to prevail in due course.

AMP are right to insist that QALYs do not at present properly measure the benefits derived from the full range of available medical therapies. They are correct in pointing out that current systems of clinical budgeting do not yet furnish adequate incentives for the efficient use of hospital resources. And they are justified in drawing attention to the ambiguities which weaken the present system of option appraisal for major capital expenditures. But they cannot deny that the health care system will best meet the needs of the population at large only when the medical benefits produced by the system are accurately monitored on a regular basis and when the resources devoted to health care are employed with a minimum of waste. Their study clearly shows, in my judgement, that of all those involved in the system of health care, the independent health economists are the most firmly committed to redesigning the NHS in accordance with this principle of rational action.

Furthermore, their study also shows that, despite the lapses and mistakes which are inevitable in the complex realm of practical affairs, health economists have begun to push things in the right direction. For example, option appraisal is now mandatory in the NHS for large capital expenditures, clinical budgeting is well on the way to being established, and QALYs are coming to be used as well as debated. Progress has undoubtedly been much slower than was envisaged in the euphoric, early days of health economics and the available economic techniques still need much refinement. Thus the overall impact on the operation of the NHS has, admittedly, so far been quite small. But the foundation for more rapid advance has now been laid, and given a favourable economic and political environment, there are good reasons to be optimistic about the eventual success of health economics in Britain and therefore about the long-term future of the NHS.

One further topic needs to be addressed here, namely the implications that health economics has for less-advanced areas of applied social science. As is well understood, the basic process of application is simple. In the physical sciences, careful study of the natural world has led to greater knowledge, which is then extended to applied domains in the form of technologies. The case of health economics confirms that things are much the same in the social sciences. To begin with, it shows that an applied social science must have at its disposal a powerful, widely applicable set of theoretical principles. Thus it was the availability of such a theoretical framework that enabled economists to identify the ills of the NHS and to prescribe the remedy in general outline. Second, it must be possible to provide specific, theory-based techniques, such as those derived from cost–benefit analysis, that can be employed to solve a range of particular problems. Only by means of such techniques can applied social science supply practical assistance of a concrete, useful kind. Third, the case of health economics suggests that although applied social scientists must have clear-cut, long-term objectives, they must be prepared to accept compromise and modest advance in the short run.

The fourth general implication to be drawn from health economics is that it is advisable to carry out at an early stage a careful, systematic appraisal of the scale and complexity of the overall task that has to be undertaken. If this is not done, as seems to have been the case in health economics, frustration and disappointment, cynicism and even despair, may ensue. It is in this area that British health economists have been most obviously at fault. For they have made little attempt to organize their own collective activities along rational lines. In other words, they have not applied to themselves the same criteria of adequacy that they have used to judge the operation of the NHS. Like the health service, British health economics has operated in a piecemeal and *ad hoc* fashion. It is no guarantee of the rationality of health economics that its diverse activities continue to be funded. For we have seen that doctors continue to receive their salaries despite the economic irrationality of much of their conduct. Furthermore, given the nature of the health care system, financial support for health economics may well be regularly forthcoming for services that perpetuate, rather than reduce, the current level of irrationality. Thus it is a culpable failure on the part of health economists that they have made no real attempt to devise and implement a co-ordinated programme of self-monitoring applied social science which would demonstrate that their own use of resources is efficient, that the gains in welfare arising from their activities are considerable, and that their efforts could not be better spent elsewhere.

Health economists are to be commended for entering the vanguard of applied social science in Britain. Nevertheless, we must take notice of their errors as well as their successes if we are to learn from their exploratory efforts. In particular, we must make sure that applied social scientists in other areas do not exempt themselves from the requirements of economic efficiency which are applied so stringently to non-social scientists and that, unlike the health economists studied by AMP, they build into their practice a variety of reliable mechanisms for assessing and advancing the level of their own economic rationality.

Critical deconstruction: a sociologist's reading

Pinch, Ashmore and Mulkay (PAM) have described above in some detail how the community of health economics operates within the British setting. They have shown how the members of that community have managed to formulate their expertise in a relatively modest way which has enabled them to gain access to the institutions of health care provision and to establish a relationship of interdependency. PAM's analysis in previous chapters reveals how health economists' ensuing attempts to move the NHS as a whole in what they regard as a more rational direction have met with comparatively little success; partly due to the massive scale of that organization, but even more significantly to the complexity of its internal dynamics. They have also shown how, more recently, some health economists have largely abandoned the initial strategy of reasoned argument and rational discussion and have resorted to public confrontation and the emotive rhetoric of the mass media. The general impression conveyed by PAM's analysis is that economists' prolonged contact with the supposed irrationalities of the health care system has done more to reduce the rationality of their own practices than to improve that of the NHS. In particular, PAM's detailed examination of option appraisal, clinical budgeting and QALYs, shows clearly how these rational techniques are transformed within the context of the NHS and how they become available as flexible resources in an essentially political process of decision-making.

Regrettably PAM's analysis, like much microsociology, has failed to pay sufficient attention to the wider social processes. For example, conditions were ripe during the 1970s and 1980s in Britain for the social science of health economics to make a major impact upon the British system of health care. Particular policies on the health service, as PAM themselves note, have embraced ideas drawn from health economics. Thus the Griffiths Inquiry set up by the government in 1983 was instrumental in providing a legislative push to health authorities to adopt changes in management practices and to introduce clinical and management budgeting. Also option appraisal for capital schemes was made mandatory by DHSS directive in 1982.

The indirect influences have probably been even more significant. In many areas of public life during the Thatcher years we have seen the rise of free-market economics and the celebration of the 'enterprise culture' with its attendant economic catchphrases such as 'efficiency', 'choice', 'value for money' and 'rationalization'. I do not mean to imply that all professional economists have openly endorsed the simple-minded economics of Thatcherism (although some clearly have), but it would be wrong to underestimate the effects on the general climate of opinion of a government committed to the practical implementation of such ideas as a cure for Britain's economic malaise. One of these effects is that economic concepts are no longer treated as the terminology of an alien social science, but as part of a plausible language of action. Often, we are now told, 'there is no alternative' but to move towards ever greater economic rationality. There can be no denying that economics has become increasingly entrenched in the wider political scene (*Radical Community Medicine* 1986/7), a fact which PAM have largely ignored.

This is particularly ironic given PAM's emphasis on health economists' attempts to draw a firm distinction between rational economic action, on the one hand, and politics and other forms of non-rational conduct, on the other. Economic choices are seen by health economists as taking place in a non-economic environment which can either impede or promote rationality. In the case of the NHS, the environment is regarded as overwhelmingly irrational and negative; that is, it lowers the level of economic efficiency by ensuring that much of participants' conduct is unsystematic, uninformed, based upon tacit judgements which are not open to public scrutiny, influenced by social and personal commitments, and so on. It appears that the guiding aim of health economics is to reduce the impact of such factors on the provision of health care services by establishing decision-making procedures which embody a kind of pure economic action. In other words, such procedures are taken to provide a detached, precise evaluation of means and ends which identifies those outcomes that would furnish the greatest possible benefit.

PAM show that in practice health economists constantly qualify and moderate this strong formulation of their remedial programme, but that without the strong programme they have no persuasive rationale for attempting to reform the NHS. Unless they remain committed to implementing their theory-based conception of rational action, economists' role in the health service is reduced to that of supplementary administrative workers. PAM maintain, however, that the economists' practical techniques cannot be made to work in accordance with the requirements of the strong programme. They show that the health economists' own procedures are inherently uncertain, imprecise and dependent on the kind of tacit judgements and social negotiations that are deemed, from the economists' theoretical perspective, to be irrational.

Economists, of course, frequently acknowledge that their practical solutions seldom operate perfectly. But these departures from optimality are typically seen as unfortunate, and potentially avoidable, consequences of the intrusion of temporarily uncontrolled environmental factors. PAM insist, in contrast, that evaluative contradictions, tacit judgements, variability of perspectives, conflicts of interest and social negotiations are necessary features of all social conduct, including that of the health economists. Thus PAM emphasize that they are not engaged in revealing the technical inadequacies of particular economic techniques or of individual economists. They are, rather, arguing that human practical action by its very nature does not fit into the decision-making calculus derived from economic theory and that it can be made to appear to do so only by means of 'irrational', that is, socially located, covert and contingent interpretations on the part of the technical experts themselves, which are hidden from view behind the impersonal facade of economic discourse.

PAM do not, in my view, make their own, alternative conception of social action sufficiently clear and precise. Nevertheless, there can be no doubt that PAM, like other sociologists, differ considerably from economists in their assumptions about the fundamental characteristics of human conduct. Unlike economists, PAM seem to contend that economic activity in the real world is best conceived, not as a separate realm of action amenable to definitive formulation in terms of a specialized brand of self-contained analysis, but rather as one aspect of a complex web of human interaction which is essentially multi-faceted, multi-dimensional and in constant flux. Consequently, it follows, for them, that in the everyday world of practical action, economic judgements will always be indissolubly linked to so-called non-economic factors.

Furthermore, from their sociological perspective, individuals cannot be regarded as having a given set of preferences, economic or otherwise, to which their conduct is rationally oriented. As PAM argue in their critique of QALYs, it is necessary to accept instead that actors are capable of identifying their preferences in many different, and often apparently contradictory, ways depending on the circumstances in which those preferences are being specified (Potter and Wetherell 1987). Social action, they seem to argue, is to be seen not as a clear-cut, unitary, internally consistent realm but as an essentially ambiguous, multiple, ever-changing process. As Iden Wickings (a non-economist) is quoted as saying in Chapter 6, 'There isn't a monocular view of the world is there? I mean if you have got one, you're more a fool I think'. Of course, some economists have come to somewhat similar conclusions and have challenged traditional economic theory accordingly:

> A person is given *one* preference ordering, and as and when the need arises this is supposed to reflect his interests, represent his welfare, summarize his idea of what should be done, and describe his actual choices and behaviour. Can one preference ordering do all these things? A person thus described may be 'rational' in the limited sense of revealing no inconsistencies in his choice behaviour, but if he has no use for these distinctions between quite different concepts, he must be a bit of a fool. The *purely* economic man is indeed close to being a social moron. Economic theory has been much preoccupied with this rational fool decked in the glory of his *one* all-purpose preference ordering.
>
> (Sen 1979: 102)

However, this kind of internal questioning has not altered the basic model of economic thinking which lies behind the technical practice of health economics.

If we accept that the model of the economic actor, what Sen calls the concept of the 'rational fool', is seriously inadequate when applied to the comparatively simple case of the individual person, it becomes inconceivable that it could be used to cope with the vastly more complex case of large-scale social collectivities such as the NHS or its constituent parts. Yet, if PAM are correct, this is precisely what health economists have tried to do; that is, they have attempted to treat the NHS (or an NHS region or district or hospital) analytically as a single actor whose preferences can be ranked and whose resources can be allocated accordingly. It is evident from the preceding chapters that such techniques as QALYs and option appraisal must eliminate from consideration any differences of opinion and judgement among subgroups or individuals within the analytical unit in order to produce a single, best course of action for the collective rational actor. Economists, it seems, try to represent the resulting decisions as expressions of the collectivity's preferences. However, PAM show unequivocally that these so-called preferences and the supposedly rational decisions which they generate are contingent and affected by the social context of their production. They appear to suggest that this situation cannot be regarded as that of a group of social scientists helping laypersons to identify their own best possible course of practical action, but rather that of a group of social scientists employing an unduly narrow conception of human conduct to furnish a decision-making format which gives an illusion of rationality to the socially negotiated outcomes of the administrative process.

We have seen throughout the chapters above that health economists are particularly likely to condemn as irrational what they often describe as 'political' action – that is, action that is based upon some restricted, sectional view and which is thought to further some sectional interests at the expense of other parties. PAM show clearly that health economists have been continually frustrated by what they see as the unfortunate persistence of such local social commitments on the part of participants within the health service. Yet it seems likely that socially restricted commitments, for example, to one's ward, one's medical specialism or one's hospital, are an essential part of all economic action in real world settings:

> Every economic system has . . . tended to rely on the existence of attitudes toward work which supersede the calculation of net gain from each unit of exertion . . . one reason why economists have so little to contribute in this area is the neglect in traditional economic theory of this whole issue of commitment and the social relations surrounding it.
>
> (Sen 1979: 100–1)

From a sociological perspective, Sen's point is self-evident. It is obvious, sociologically, that commitment by participants to their subgroupings is critical for the operation of any complex organization. It is equally obvious that participants' formulations of their values and preferences, their interpretations of the organization to which they belong, and their assessments of its outcomes will all be influenced by, and to some degree moulded by, their social location. This means, for example, that participants' views of the operation of the NHS are unavoidably diverse and discrepant, due to the very nature of its internal organization as well as to the variety of its members' external obligations. From the economists' theoretical perspective, participants' sectional interests, interpretations and evaluations are to be dismissed as partial and as politically, that is, socially, engendered. It is evident, however, that practitioners' views are seen by economists as partial and biased precisely because, and in so far as, they do not coincide with the results of the economists' technical manipulations. Yet it was noted in the discussion of QALYs in Chapter 5 that the economists' conclusions will only occasionally, by chance, converge with those of any subsection of participants. Thus the great majority of participants are doomed to the charge of irrationality by the very nature of the economists' procedures. Moreover, if we focus upon the health economists' own practical actions, we find that they are no more free from the influence of group membership and sectional perspective than those of anyone else. In other words, from the sociological viewpoint, the economists' contribution to the health care system is but one more partial, socially located input, derived ultimately from the limited cultural resources of academic economics. The economists' claim to have privileged access to rationality in practical affairs is seen to be an artefact of their peculiar model of social action and of the practical techniques to which this model gives rise. It seems to follow that, when viewed sociologically, health economists stand on an equal footing with other participants and that their practical usefulness is properly to be judged, not by their own restricted standards, but in accordance with other parties' perspectives and commitments.

This seems to me to be the main practical message of PAM's analysis of health economics. On this reading, PAM may be seen as endorsing a version of the economists' own weak programme. But the general implications of their study go well beyond this. For PAM are clearly asserting that there cannot be a single valid account of the operation of the NHS or of any other complex social organization. It is for this reason, presumably, that their text employs several different presentational formats which allow into the analysis a variety of discrepant voices, each of which appears to speak from a different social location and each of which interprets the NHS in its own distinctive way. Such an approach may be adequate, like the economists' model of the rational actor, for purposes of academic analysis. It certainly appears to give the sociologists committed to this view the unique ability to encompass every possible perspective on the social world. In this respect, PAM seem to out-do the economists in claiming to adopt a wider view and in maintaining that they represent the community at large. PAM's notion of applied social science is apparently drawn from recent work in the sociology of science (Bijker, Hughes and Pinch 1987). Rather than treating application as the straightforward extension of a body of knowledge to a new domain, they claim that health economics, like other sciences, is transformed and redefined in the very process of application: for PAM, this is how the 'science of choice' becomes the 'rationalized choice'. But, in my view, it is doubtful whether their relativistic version of sociology, which insists on the social production of all versions of the world including their own, can ever provide the basis for an effective form of applied social science. For if analysts refuse to treat their own accounts as interpretatively privileged, they will be unable to assess social life in a critical fashion and will be unable to indicate how specific improvements could be brought about.

There is, therefore, a contradiction or paradox at the heart of PAM's approach to sociological analysis and to applied social science. We may call this the 'paradox of applied relativism'. At one level, their analysis leaves their subjects untouched, despite its superficially critical tone. For instance, PAM accept that health economists need both the strong and the weak programmes and that, although health economics is but one limited subculture among many, it could not, in principle, be otherwise. This may be said to follow from PAM's own weak programme. Yet at a more fundamental level, PAM are accusing economists of employing an inadequate conception of social action and, consequently, of devising a form of applied social science which fails to cope with the multiplicity of the social world. Thus PAM also supply a strong programme which implicitly urges all social scientists to adopt *their* conception of social action and to use *their* kind of new literary forms as a way of giving textual space to alternative voices and presumably, in the long run, as a way of allowing non-social scientists a more active role in forming the recommendations of applied social science.

The paradox is, of course, that PAM's strong programme requires them to claim a privileged status for their own model of social action and their own textual practices. In criticizing an applied social science for not adopting their perspective, they are undoubtedly involved, no matter how much they deny it, in asserting their own practical as well as analytical superiority. Like the health economists, PAM seem to employ both a strong and a weak programme, between which they move in a flexible manner. I am not sure whether this disproves, or confirms, their analysis.

Sceptical self-realization: a layperson's reading

It's very nice of these social scientists to let me have a say. I'll do my best to help them. They seem to be in quite a muddle. But they have studied these things much more than me and if they can't work things out on their own, I'm not sure that I can be of any great assistance. In fact, I'm rather surprised to be given this chance to participate, because I noticed that they seem to be much more interested in each other than in people like me. For example, first the economists criticized the doctors and the NHS administrators and showed them where they'd gone wrong. Then the sociologists came along and criticized the economists. I suppose I could have a go at telling the sociologists where *they* are mistaken. However, the other sociologist who wrote the previous ending has already done that. He seemed pretty convincing. But then they all do to begin with – until you ask what it means for ordinary people in practical terms.

I was upset by that dismissive reference in Chapter 5 about writing 'chatty biographies concerning Mrs Jones and then generalizing to the country at large', or something like that. Well, I *am* Mrs Jones, and I object to being condensed into a set of statistics. I'm well aware that my experiences and expectations of the health service won't be the same as other people's. But this seems to me a good reason for trying to take our different views into account instead of ignoring them. I realize that that sounds like a tall order. The administrators will ask: how can we deal personally with 50 million unique individuals? And of course, they're right. It can't be done. But does it follow that they should turn instead to the social science experts and pay them to speak on our behalf or to allocate resources in ways which are supposed to reflect our hidden preferences? I don't think that it does. As I understand it, social scientists differ among themselves just as much as the rest of us. What seems to me to follow from economics is that, once they're being paid for their services, they will tend to avoid disrupting the present system too radically. But perhaps I've misunderstood.

Nevertheless, the more I think about it, the more I believe that we, that is, the Mrs Jones's of this world, have been increasingly prevented from actively creating our own lives by the combined operation of large-scale administration and the application of the traditional models of social science. (I'd better be careful, I'm beginning to write like a social scientist myself. On the other hand, I've got to try to speak their language in order to communicate with them.) Both administrators and social scientists, as far as I can tell from my own experience and from reading this book, treat ordinary people in the same depersonalized, exploitative way. We're always on the receiving end. We're treated as passive recipients of whatever they decide to give us. We're never given the chance to participate actively in their deliberations on our behalf. Consequently, we have lost the ability to speak to them in ways that they can understand and they have lost the ability to listen to us. The end result is that it seems on the surface to be true that we have little to offer in relation to the complex administrative problems of our times. However, I insist that this seems to be the case largely because we have been persistently denied a proper voice in the past and because both parties normally take for granted that successful communication on equal terms is impossible and not worth pursuing.

As far as the NHS is concerned, I can see no reason why people like me could not be actively involved in its operation and its decision-making at all levels. It's normally assumed in hospitals, for example, that patients are quite incapable of reasoned thought. Yet, if you've been a patient in a large ward for any length of time, you will be aware that patients are quite capable of bringing their experiences together to protest at the way the ward, and other parts of the hospital, are run. Such criticisms don't make artificial distinctions between economic and other factors. They deal concretely with the social life of the ward in its full detail and, in my opinion, they often provide suggestions for improvement which are worthy of serious consideration. But, of course, dialogue between the experts and the layperson on such matters is strictly forbidden. Thus we learn to keep quiet and the expert becomes further convinced of our apathy and incompetence.

There are many specific areas of medical treatment where more open dialogue could be beneficial to all concerned. Take the treatment of diabetes, for example. Clearly the doctor has much to give to the person suffering from this condition. Basically, she uses her knowledge to offer the patient the possibility of a reasonably normal existence in place of slow poisoning and death. Yet the individual diabetic also builds up a body of personal knowledge about the complexities and subtleties of living the diabetic life. This knowledge is not available to the doctor without the patient's help (except for the odd case where the doctor is also a diabetic). But doctors, on the whole, are uninterested in developing a reciprocal relationship with their 'non-expert' patients and the latters' knowledge and personal experience remain untapped. What I am trying to say, therefore, is that it might be possible to produce considerable improvements in patients', and doctors', welfare (using much the same economic resources) by lowering the barrier between 'expert' and 'non-expert', and by enabling ordinary people on both sides of that barrier to learn from each other.

I could write at considerable length about the provision of medical services because my family and I have had much experience of the NHS. But I think that I have made my main point; which is, that the introduction of more give-and-take into the relations between patients and doctors would probably make good economic, as well as social, sense. My direct experience of social science is, in contrast, much more limited. However, I have read the chapters above with some care and I certainly don't like the idea of being thought of as a 'rational fool'. Nor do I think that those economics professors had any right to claim to be representing *my* wishes when they advised the NHS to reduce support for kidney dialysis in favour of hip replacements. In my opinion, it would be much better to spend less money on those infuriating RAF aeroplanes that scream around the countryside preparing for a Russian invasion and increase treatment both for hips *and* for kidneys. So I think that those sociologists, AMP, or perhaps it's PAM, are probably on the right lines when they criticize the economists.

Yet I'm not sure that they have anything better to offer. I got the impression that they were in favour of changing sociology so that the so-called expert's voice didn't dominate so much. I certainly approve of *that*. But of *course* I approve! I'm no more than a textual device of their making. I'm entirely under their control. It seems to me that I'm rather like the economists' rhetoric of rationality, behind which they exercise their own hidden judgements. I'm an illusion of multivocality (that word is clumsy enough to sound like social science), behind which the sociologists continue to assume their own privileged knowledge of the social world. So I think we need one more paradox: that social scientists can only claim to speak on our behalf by refusing to let us speak for ourselves. I think we'll call this the 'paradox of applied social science'.

Appendix: Research materials

Interviews and transcripts

During the period of research (October 1985 to July 1988) we conducted a total of sixty-five interviews with sixty-nine interviewees, a few being interviewed jointly. The interviews took place from January to April 1986, December 1986 to March 1987 and in March 1988. The interviewees can be categorized as follows:

- Thirty-six outsiders (health economists working in an academic context).
- Eight insiders (health economists working within the health service).
- Fourteen practitioners (non-economists working within the health service).
- Nine critics (academic critics of health economics).
- Two evaluators (members of the clinical budgeting Evaluation Group – see Ch. 6).

Of the outsiders, twelve were based at the Centre for Health Economics, University of York; ten at the Health Economics Research Unit, University of Aberdeen; five at the Health Economics Research Group, Brunel University, and nine elsewhere. Of the insiders, only one worked officially as a health economist. The others worked variously in Health Authority departments of planning or finance or in the DHSS. Among the practitioners, ten were clinicians and four were administrators. The academic backgrounds of the critics were economics (three), sociology (two), medical statistics (two), management (one) and philosophy (one).

The interviews, which lasted from twenty minutes to three hours, were usually carried out by a pair of authors using the semi-structured format of a schedule of topics and analytical issues formulated for each category of interviewee supplemented in most cases by a set of specific questions arising out of our prior knowledge of the work of the participant concerned. As an illustration, here is our 'Health Practitioners' Interview Outline':

(A) Outline of interview:
Questions on your career, technical questions about your work, your connections with health economics (HE) and health economists, and questions on the application of HE in practice.

(B) Career questions:
Give brief summary (if known).
or Ask for brief summary.
- (1) Institutions attended.
- (2) Subjects studied.
- (3) Manner of entry into job.
- (4) Listing of projects and involvement:
  - (a) Main 'themes' of career
  - (b) Current interests
  - (c) Current problems
  - (d) Future plans
- (5) 'Standard week' description.
- (6) Relation of work to HE.

(Emphasis on academic/practical movements)

(C) 'Your work': technical questions.

(D) Application of HE: costs and benefits.
- (1) Relations with health economists:
  Problems?
  Of what kind?
- (2) Resistance to HE by health practitioners:
  Much?
  Little?
  On what grounds?
  Which practitioner groups (doctors, nurses, administrators, trade unions) more than others?
- (3) Is 'good' HE best done by academics (or: in an academic setting) or by practitioners (or: in a practical setting)?
  With or without specific practical goals?
- (4) Which HE research has been most successfully applied (to your knowledge)?
  How?

By whom? In what context?
With what outcome?
Which HE research has been most *un*successfully applied?
Why?
In what context?
With what result?
What is the criterion of 'success' here?

(5) How far has HE helped you to achieve your own goals?
Has it had the effect of changing those goals?

(6) Is HE a set of techniques? and/or
is HE a specific way of thinking?
If so, what are they? / what is it?

(7) Does the application of HE imply a particular view of the world / set of values / desired outcome?

(8) Conflicts and oppositions:
(a) Effectiveness (medical) v efficiency (economic)
(b) Economics v ethics
(c) Medical science (priority?) v economic science
(d) Efficiency v equity.

(9) Measurement:
What can be measured?
What cannot be measured?
Technical reason?
Fundamental (impossibility) reason?

(10) Money:
Necessary aspect of HE work? Costs, etc.?
or only convenient (technical) measuring-rod?

(11) Rationality – 'Economic man' a reality or a fiction?

(12) Politics of health service:
HE contribution (which side are they on?)
Helps or hinders successful HE application?

(E) Economics and Science.

(1) Definition of economics?
(2) Is economics a science?
Is [your academic discipline, if one claimed] a science?
What kind?
Like physics, mathematics, sociology, medicine — differences and distinctions?
(3) Is HE an application of 'economics' to 'health'?
(4) Distinctions/differences between economics and accountancy.

All except one of the interviews were tape-recorded and transcribed verbatim. The transcripts were 'coded' by reading them with reference to our developing lists of 'participants' topics', such as option appraisal or QALYs, and 'analytical topics', such as rationality or 'quick and dirty'. Each topic was allocated an index card and every time a topic was addressed in a transcript the interviewee's name together with the page number was entered on the card. In this way we built up a continually updated file of relevant extracts.

Texts

The texts which we collected, read, discussed and transformed during the course of the study include health economists' academic books and articles, their critics' publications, the series of discussion papers issued by the major British centres of health economics, Health Economists' Study Group conference papers, various seminar papers, relevant government publications, documents issued at press conferences, articles in the medical and general press by and about health economists, internal health authority reports and documentation, the main research centres' publicity material (CHE's *Newsletter*, HERU's *Bulletin*, YHEC's *Monitor*), and, from members of the Centre at York, a selection of their CVs, teaching materials, research proposals, research reports and internal memoranda.

Recorded events

We recorded, on audiotape and sometimes videotape, health economists talking in the following lectures, seminars, conferences, courses and meetings:

RCN, BMA and IHSM Press Conference, London, 30 October 1985 (video).
Economics Society Lecture, York, 30 October 1985 (video).
Health Economists' Policy Group meeting, York, 5 November 1985.
Centre for Health Economics seminars, York, 5 December 1985, 29 January 1986, 13 June 1986.
Health Economists' Study Group conferences, York, 8–10 January 1986 and Bath, 7–9 July 1986.
'Effectiveness and Efficiency in Patient Care: A Course for Clinicians', Bowness-on-Windermere, Cumbria, 17–18 March 1986 (video).
British Association for the Advancement of Science, Economics section lectures, Bristol, 2 September 1986.

'Medical Ethics and Economics' conference, Lisse, the Netherlands, 24–6 September 1986.
NHS Health Economics Group meeting, York, 1 July 1987.

We also recorded three television programmes and three radio broadcasts in which health economists took part:

Heart of the Matter, BBC1, 7 October 1986.
This Week, ITV, 9 October 1986.
This Week, ITV, 16 October 1986.
Medicine Now, BBC Radio 4, 11 December 1986.
Today, BBC Radio 4, 15 December 1987.
International Assignment, BBC Radio 4, 15 January 1988.

Finally, we recorded most of the talks we gave to health economists and others about our work as well as a series of project discussions which took place during the early phases of the research.

Bibliography

Alban, A. (1982). 'Economic appraisal: what is the use?' Presented at the Third Nordic Health Economists' Study Group meeting, Oslo, September 1982.

Akehurst, R.L. (1986). *Planning Hospital Services: An Option Appraisal of a Major Health Service Rationalisation.* University of York, Centre for Health Economics Discussion Paper, 12.

——(1987). 'Economic appraisal applied to health care planning: some reflections on the use of option appraisal in the NHS'. Presented to the Health Economists' Study Group/Institute of Health Service Managers Conference, University of York, July 1987.

Akehurst, R.L. and M.J. Buxton (1985). 'Option appraisal in the NHS: a guide to better decision-making'. *Nuffield/York Portfolios* 8: 1–4. London, Nuffield Provincial Hospitals Trust.

Akehurst, R.L. and S. Holtermann (1985). *Provision of Decentralised Mental Illness Services: An Option Appraisal.* University of York, Centre for Health Economics Discussion Paper, 5.

Ashmore, M. (1988). 'The life and opinions of a replication claim: reflexivity and symmetry in the sociology of scientific knowledge'. In S. Woolgar (ed.), *Knowledge and Reflexivity: New Frontiers in the Sociology of Knowledge.* London and Beverly Hills, Sage Publications.

——(1989). *The Reflexive Thesis: Wrighting Sociology of Scientific Knowledge.* Chicago and London, University of Chicago Press.

Ashmore, M., M.J. Mulkay, T.J. Pinch and HESG (1988). 'Definitional work in applied social science: collaborative analysis in health economics and sociology of science'. In L. Hargens, R.A. Jones and A. Pickering (eds.), *Knowledge and Society*, vol. 8. Greenwich, Conn., JAI Press.

Ashmore, M., T.J. Pinch and M.J. Mulkay (1987). 'The rationalized choice: an examination of an option appraisal'. Typescript, University of York.

Atkinson, M. (1984). *Our Masters' Voices: The Language and Body Language of Politics*. London and New York, Methuen.

Bevan, G. (1984). 'The structure of the National Health Service'. In N. Black, D. Boswell, A. Gray, S. Murphy and J. Popay (eds.), *Health and Disease: A Reader*. Milton Keynes, Open University Press.

Bijker, W., T.P. Hughes and T.J. Pinch (eds.) (1987). *The Social Construction of Technological Systems: New Directions in the Sociology and History of Technology*. Cambridge, Mass., MIT Press.

Bloor, D. (1976). *Knowledge and Social Imagery*. London, Routledge & Kegan Paul.

Burchell, A. and B.K. Gilbert (1982). *Appraisal of Development Options in the National Health Service*. London, DHSS.

Chubin, D.E. and S. Restivo (1983). 'The "mooting" of science studies: research programmes and science policy'. In K.D. Knorr-Cetina and M.J. Mulkay (eds.), *Science Observed: Perspectives on the Social Study of Science*. London and Beverly Hills, Sage Publications.

Cicourel, A. (1964). *Method and Measurement in Sociology*. New York, Free Press.

Collins, H.M. (1985). *Changing Order: Replication and Induction in Scientific Practice*. London and Beverly Hills, Sage Publications.

——(1988). 'Public experiments and displays of virtuosity: the core-set revisited'. *Social Studies of Science* 18: 725–48.

Collins, H.M. and T.J. Pinch (1979). 'Constructing the paranormal: nothing unscientific is happening'. In R. Wallis (ed.), *On the Margins of Science: The Social Construction of Rejected Knowledge, Sociological Review Monograph* 27. Keele, Keele University Press.

——(1982). *Frames of Meaning: The Social Construction of Extraordinary Science*. London, Routledge & Kegan Paul.

Colvin, P. (1985). *The Economic Ideal in British Government: Calculating Costs and Benefits in the 1970s*. Manchester, Manchester University Press.

Constant, E.W., II. (1980). *The Origins of the Turbojet Revolution*. Baltimore, Md., Johns Hopkins University Press.

Cooper, M. and A.J. Culyer (eds.) (1973). *Health Economics*. Harmondsworth, Penguin Books.

Culyer, A.J. (1976). *Need and the National Health Service: Economics and Social Choice*. Oxford, Martin Robertson.

——(1981). 'Health, economics and health economics'. In J. Van der Gaag and M. Perlman (eds.), *Health, Economics and Health Economics*. Amsterdam, North-Holland.

——(1984). 'The quest for efficiency in the public sector: economists versus Dr Pangloss'. In *Public Finance and the Quest for Efficiency*. Proceedings of the 38th Congress of the International Institute of Public Finance. Detroit, Wayne State University Press.

——(1985a). Editorial. *Nuffield/York Portfolios* 10: 1. London, Nuffield Provincial Hospitals Trust.

——(1985b). *Health Service Efficiency: Appraising the Appraisers*. University of York, Centre for Health Economics Discussion Paper, 10.

——(1985c). 'A health economist on medical sociology: reflections by an unreconstructed reductionist'. *Social Science and Medicine* 20(10): 1013–21.

——(1986). 'Health economics: the topic and the discipline'. Typescript, University of York.

Denzin, N. (ed.) (1970). *Sociological Methods: A Sourcebook*. Chicago, Aldine.

——(1978). *The Research Act*. New York, McGraw Hill.

Department of Health and Social Security (1981a). *Health Notice HN(81)30*. London, DHSS.

——(1981b). *National Health Service, Review of Capricode: Building Strategy*. London, DHSS.

——(1987a). *Option Appraisal: A Guide for the National Health Service*. London, DHSS.

——(1987b). *Health Building Schemes: Approval in Principle. AIP Bulletin*, 1. London, DHSS.

Dowson, S. and A. Maynard (1985). 'General practice'. In A. Harrison and J. Gretton (eds.), *Health Care UK 1985: An Economic, Social and Policy Audit*. London, Policy Journals.

Drummond, M.F. (1986). 'Resource allocation decisions in health care: a role for quality of life assessments'. Typescript, Health Services Management Centre, University of Birmingham.

Engleman, S.R. (1980). 'Health economics, health economists and the NHS'. *Community Medicine* 2: 126–34.

Gabbay, J. (1985/6). 'The health economists' tool kit: towards a partial analysis'. *Radical Community Medicine*, winter: 10–13.

Gilbert, G.N. and M.J. Mulkay (1984). *Opening Pandora's Box: A Sociological Analysis of Scientists' Discourse*. Cambridge, Cambridge University Press.

Gudex, C. (1986). *QALYs and Their Use by the Health Service*. University of York, Centre for Health Economics Discussion Paper, 20.

Henderson, J. (1984). *Appraising Options*. University of Aberdeen, Health Economics Research Unit, Series of Option Appraisal Papers, 2.

Henderson, J., N. Cumming, L. Kilpatrick, D. McKenzie and M. Stirling (1985). *Mental Handicap Beds for Dumfries and Galloway*. University of Aberdeen, Health Economics Research Unit, Series of Option Appraisal Papers, 7.

Henderson, J., A. McGuire and D. Parkin (1984a). *Acute Hospital Beds for Fife: 1, Appraisal of Options.* University of Aberdeen, Health Economics Research Unit, Series of Option Appraisal Papers, 3.

——(1984b). *Acute Hospital Beds for Fife: 2, Using Economics in Health Service Planning.* University of Aberdeen, Health Economics Research Unit, Series of Option Appraisal Papers, 5.

Henderson, J. and G.H. Mooney (1984). *Economic Principles of Applied Option Appraisal.* University of Aberdeen, Health Economics Research Unit, Series of Option Appraisal Papers, 1.

Holton, G. (1978). *The Scientific Imagination: Case Studies.* Cambridge, Cambridge University Press.

Kind, P., R. Rosser and A. Williams (1982). 'Valuation of quality of life: some psychometric evidence'. In M.W. Jones-Lee (ed.), *The Value of Life and Safety.* Amsterdam, North-Holland.

Klarman, H.E. (1965). *The Economics of Health.* London and New York, Columbia University Press.

Knorr-Cetina, K.D. and M.J. Mulkay (eds.) (1983). *Science Observed: Perspectives on the Social Study of Science.* London and Beverly Hills, Sage Publications.

Latour, B. (1983). 'Give me a laboratory and I will raise the world'. In K.D. Knorr-Cetina and M.J. Mulkay (eds.), *Science Observed: Perspectives on the Social Study of Science.* London and Beverly Hills, Sage Publications.

——(1987). *Science in Action: How to Follow Scientists and Engineers Through Society.* Milton Keynes, Open University Press.

Latour, B. and S. Woolgar (1979). *Laboratory Life: The Social Construction of Scientific Facts.* London and Beverly Hills, Sage Publications; 2nd edn, Princeton, NJ, Princeton University Press, 1986.

Lee, K. and A. Mills (1979). 'The role of economists and economics in health service planning: a general overview'. In K. Lee (ed.), *Economics and Health Planning.* Beckenham, Croom Helm.

Ludbrook, A. (1984). *Economic Appraisal in the NHS: A Survey.* University of Aberdeen, Health Economics Research Unit Discussion Paper, 01/84.

Ludbrook, A. and G.H. Mooney (1984). *Economic Appraisal in the NHS: Problems and Challenges.* Aberdeen, Northern Health Economics Publications.

McCloskey, D.N. (1985) *The Rhetoric of Economics.* Madison, Wis., University of Wisconsin Press.

MacKenzie, D. (1988). 'From Kwajalein to Armageddon? Testing and the social construction of missile accuracy'. In D. Gooding, T.J.

Pinch and S. Schaffer (eds.), *The Uses of Experiment: Studies of Experiment in the Natural Sciences.* Cambridge, Cambridge University Press.

Maynard, A. (1986). 'Policy choices in the health sector'. In R. Berthoud (ed.), *Challenges to Social Policy.* London, Policy Studies Institute.

Milgram, S. (1963). 'Behavioral study of obedience'. *Journal of Abnormal Social Psychology* 67: 371–8.

——(1974). *Obedience to Authority: An Experimental View.* New York, Harper & Row.

Mooney, G.H. and M.F. Drummond (1982, 1983). *The Essentials of Health Economics.* (12 articles published in 6 parts.)

Part I. 'What is economics?' *British Medical Journal (BMJ)* 285 (2 October 1982): 949–50, and (9 October): 1024–5.

Part II. 'Financing health care'. *BMJ* 285 (16 October): 1101–2, and (23 October): 1191–2.

Part III. 'Developing health care policies'. *BMJ* 285 (30 October): 1263–4, and (6 November): 1329–31.

Part IV. 'Organizing health care resources'. *BMJ* 285 (13 November): 1405–6, and (20 November): 1485–6.

Part V. 'Assessing the costs and benefits of treatment alternatives'. *BMJ* 285 (27 November): 1561–3, and (4 December): 1638–9.

Part VI. 'Challenges for the future'. *BMJ* 285 (11 December): 1727–8, and *BMJ* 286 (1 January 1983): 40–1.

Mooney, G.H. and J. Henderson (1984). *Option Appraisal in the NHS: The Road to Efficiency*? University of Aberdeen, Health Economics Research Unit Discussion Paper, 10/84.

Mulkay, M.J. (1984). 'The scientist talks back: a one-Act play, with a moral, about replication in science and reflexivity in sociology'. *Social Studies of Science* 14: 265–82.

——(1985). *The Word and the World: Explorations in the Form of Sociological Analysis.* London, George Allen & Unwin.

Mulkay, M.J., M. Ashmore, and T.J. Pinch, (1987). 'Measuring the quality of life: a sociological invention concerning the application of economics to health care'. *Sociology* 21: 541–64.

Pinch, T.J. (1986). *Confronting Nature: The Sociology of Solar-Neutrino Detection.* Dordrecht and Boston, Reidel.

Pinch, T.J., M. Ashmore and M.J. Mulkay (1987). 'Social technologies: to test or not to test, that is the question'. Presented to the International Workshop on the Integration of Social and Historical Studies of Technology, University of Twente, the Netherlands, September 1987.

Pinch, T.J. and T.J. Pinch (1988). 'Reservations about reflexivity and new literary forms: or why let the Devil have all the good tunes?' In S. Woolgar (ed.), *Knowledge and Reflexivity: New Frontiers in the*

Sociology of Knowledge. London and Beverly Hills, Sage Publications.

Potter, J. and M. Wetherell (1987). *Discourse and Social Psychology: Beyond Attitudes and Behaviour*. London and Beverly Hills, Sage Publications.

Radical Community Medicine (1986/7). Special issue on 'The economics of health'. Winter.

Rosser, R. and P. Kind (1978). 'A scale of valuations of states of illness'. *International Journal of Epidemiology* 7: 347–58.

Schutz, A. (1972). *The Phenomenology of the Social World*. London, Heinemann.

Sen, A.K. (1979). 'Rational fools'. In F. Hahn and M. Hollis (eds.), *Philosophy and Economic Theory*. Oxford, Oxford University Press.

Strong, P.M. (1979). 'Sociological imperialism and the profession of medicine: a critical examination of the thesis of medical imperialism'. *Social Science and Medicine* 13A: 199–215.

——(1985/6). 'The economists' contribution to health policy: the view from another social science'. *Radical Community Medicine*, winter: 7–10.

Thunhurst, C. (1985/6). 'Close encounters of an economic kind'. *Radical Community Medicine*, winter: 18–26.

Treasury (1982, 1984). *Investment Appraisal in the Public Sector*. London, HMSO.

West, P. (1985/6). 'Too many economists?' *Radical Community Medicine*, winter: 13–17.

——(1986). 'Clinical budgeting: a critique'. Presented at the Health Economists' Study Group Meeting, University of Bath, July 1986.

West, P., G.H. Mooney and R. Trevillion (1984). 'Rationalisation of acute hospital services in Lewisham and North Southwark'. University of Aberdeen, Health Economics Research Unit, Series of Option Appraisal Papers, 4.

Whitley, R. (1986). 'The structure and context of economics as a scientific field'. *Research in the History of Economic Thought and Methodology* 4: 179–209.

Wickings, I. (1983). 'Griffiths Report: consultants face the figures'. *Health and Social Service Journal*, 8 December: 1466–8.

Wickings, I., T. Childs, J. Coles and C. Wheatcroft (1985). *Experiments Using PACTs in Southend and Oldham HAs*. CASPE research report, CASPE, King's Fund, London.

Wickings, I. and Coles, J. (1985). 'The ethical imperative of clinical budgeting'. *Nuffield/York Portfolios* 10: 1–8. London, Nuffield Provincial Hospitals Trust.

Williams, A. (1972). 'Cost–benefit analysis: bastard science? and/or insidious poison in the body politick?' *Journal of Public Economics* 1: 199–225.

——(1981). 'Welfare economics and health status measurement'. In J. Van der Gaag and M. Perlman (eds.), *Health, Economics and Health Economics.* Amsterdam, North-Holland.

——(1985). 'Economics of coronary artery bypass grafting'. *British Medical Journal* 291 (3 August): 326–9.

——(1987). 'Measuring quality of life: a comment'. *Sociology* 21: 565–6.

Woolgar, S. (ed.) (1988). *Knowledge and Reflexivity: New Frontiers in the Sociology of Knowledge.* London and Beverly Hills, Sage Publications.

Yule, B. (ed.) (1987). *HEART: Health Economists' Activities, Research and Teaching*, 4, January. University of Aberdeen, Health Economics Research Unit.

Yule, B. and D. Cohen (1985). *Appraising Laundry Services in Fife: Money for Old SOAP?* University of Aberdeen, Health Economics Research Unit, Series of Option Appraisal Papers, 8.

Index